FIBROMYALGIA
freedom!

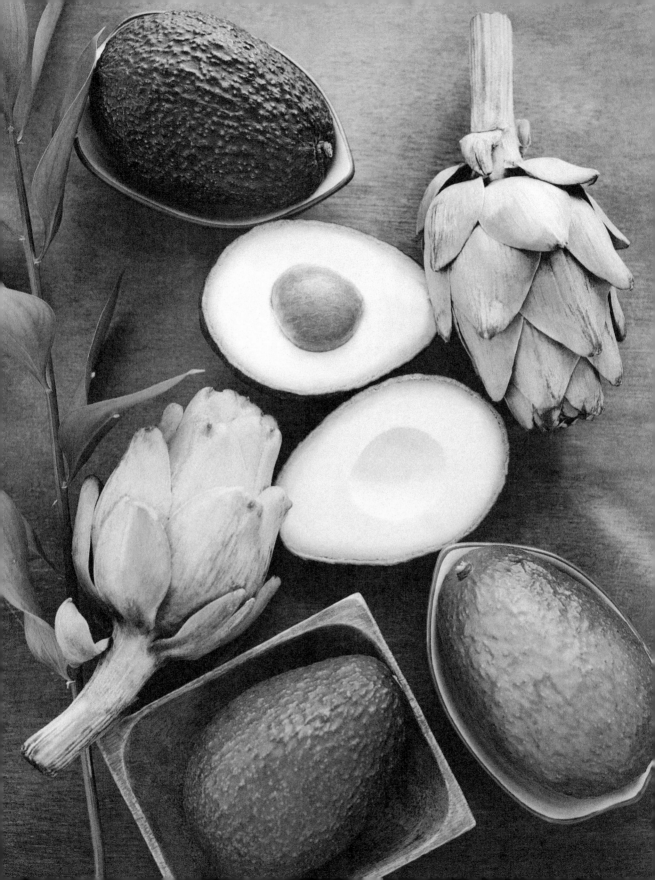

FIBROMYALGIA

freedom!

Your Essential Cookbook and Meal Plan to Relieve Pain, Clear Brain Fog & Fight Fatigue

KATHLEEN STANDAFER, RD

ROCKRIDGE
PRESS

For general information on our other products and services or to obtain technical support, please contact our Customer Care Department within the U.S. at (866) 744-2665, or outside the U.S. at (510) 253-0500.

Rockridge Press publishes its books in a variety of electronic and print formats. Some content that appears in print may not be available in electronic books, and vice versa.

Design by Kathleen Lynch and Eve Siegel

Cover Photography © Shannon Douglas
Back Cover: The Picture Pantry/Stockfood
Interior: People Pictures/Stockfood, p.ii; The Picture Pantry/Stockfood, p.vi; Dobránska Renáta/Stocksy, p.ix; Ruth Black/Stocksy, p.xii; Alberto Bogo/Stocksy, p.2; The Picture Pantry/Stockfood, p.12; Raymond Forbes LLC/Stocksy, p.22; Gräfe & Unzer Verlag/Jörn Rynio/Stockfood, p.24; Gräfe & Unzer Verlag/Fotos mit Geschmack/Stockfood, p.46; Ina Peters/Stockfood, p.60; Victoria Firmston/Stockfood, p.62; Aniko Takacs/Stockfood, p.80; Rua Castilho/Stockfood, p.100; Gräfe & Unzer Verlag/Jörn Rynio/Stockfood, p.122; Gräfe & Unzer Verlag/Jörn Rynio/Stockfood, p.136; Gräfe & Unzer Verlag/Kramp + Gölling/Stockfood, p.164; Tanya Zouev/Stockfood, p.192; Gräfe & Unzer Verlag/René Riis/Stockfood, p.202; Helen Rushbrook/Stocksy, p.216

ISBN: Print 978-1-62315-914-6 | eBook 978-1-62315-915-3

quick start guide

Your Journey to a Pain-Free Life

If you're newly diagnosed with fibromyalgia, here are five tips to get you started right away on mitigating pain and feeling better.

Practice Mindfulness. Irregular breathing and anxious thoughts can contribute to your pain. Paying close attention to your thoughts and keeping them positive and calming is a step in the right direction. A few things that can help you stay positive: Avoid over-watching the news or violent movies. Laugh as often as you can, whether it's from funny books, movies, or a dear friend who knows just what to say to get you laughing. Go for walks, enjoy the outdoors, and practice meditation or deep breathing several times throughout the day.

Boost Nutrients. Chronic pain is often exacerbated by an imbalance of nutrients. One way to ensure you're getting the right nutrients is to eat a colorful variety of whole foods, and include a vegetable, healthy fat, and protein with every meal.

Kitchen Makeover. Eliminating processed foods from your diet is one of the best ways to fight chronic pain. Get these out of your pantry, and fill your kitchen with real food. A little bit of planning can go a long way toward alleviating pain.

Honor Your Natural Circadian Rhythms. Sleep is a major factor in fibromyalgia management. Practice good sleep hygiene by eliminating screen time one hour before bedtime, making your bedroom pitch-dark, and getting some sunlight at midday every day.

Enhance Your Movement. Anytime you're not sitting, you're helping your body fight chronic pain. Stretch every morning for a few minutes when you get out of bed. Make sure you have comfortable shoes and move as much as possible throughout the day.

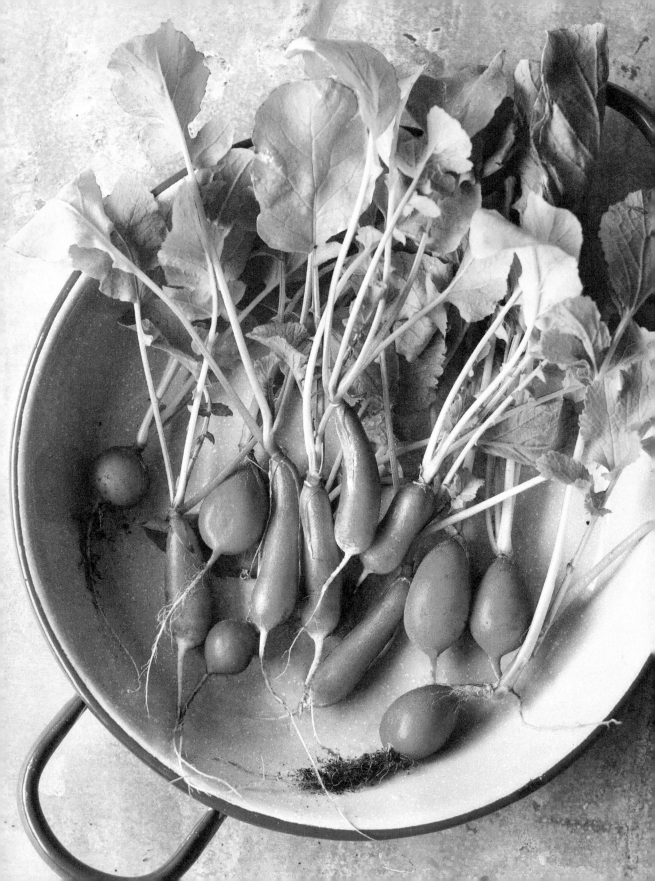

contents

Introduction viii

➣ **PART 1 BREAK UP WITH PAIN** 1

CHAPTER 1 UNDERSTANDING FIBROMYALGIA 3

CHAPTER 2 FOOD & MOVEMENT 13

➣ **PART 2 THE PLAN** 23

CHAPTER 3 FOUR WEEKS TO FIBRO FREEDOM! 25

CHAPTER 4 MEAL PLANS 47

➣ **PART 3 THE RECIPES** 61

CHAPTER 5 SMOOTHIES & BREAKFASTS 63

CHAPTER 6 SOUPS & SALADS 81

CHAPTER 7 SNACKS & SIDES 101

CHAPTER 8 VEGETARIAN & VEGAN ENTRÉES 123

CHAPTER 9 FISH & SEAFOOD ENTRÉES 137

CHAPTER 10 MEAT & POULTRY ENTRÉES 165

CHAPTER 11 DESSERTS 193

CHAPTER 12 STAPLES: BROTHS, SAUCES, & CONDIMENTS 203

Appendix A: Measurement Conversions 217

Appendix B: The Dirty Dozen & The Clean Fifteen 218

Resources 219 / References 220

Recipe Index 223 / Index 225

introduction

If you're one of the five million Americans suffering from fibromyalgia, you know what a frustrating condition it can be. But you aren't alone, and there is a lot you can do today that will put you on the path to some relief.

When I first started working as a dietitian, I treated hundreds of patients suffering from the same cluster of symptoms: widespread pain, brain fog, fatigue, and gastrointestinal discomfort. Despite their exercising and making dietary changes, symptoms waxed and waned without explanation. For many of my patients, living a normal life without pain was just a faraway memory. Other doctors dismissed their symptoms as typical problems post-menopausal women experience. On top of that, patients often blamed themselves, wondering if they were not making enough of an effort with their diet changes and exercise. This led them to either give up completely or try even more drastic measures, only to become more depressed and fatigued when those measures failed as well. It wasn't until I did more research on these symptoms and sought out specialists that I understood that the syndrome they all suffered from was fibromyalgia.

Fibromyalgia can be triggered by intense stress (including poor nutrition) if the right genes are present. The result of this stress that fibromites (what fibromyalgia sufferers call themselves) experience leads to an oversensitive central nervous system and disorders in the pathways that process pain. This scenario can be exacerbated by nutrient imbalances from eating the standard American diet (SAD; high in inflammatory fats, carbohydrates, sugar, and food additives), side effects of medications (those diagnosed with fibromyalgia often have accompanying conditions—medical diseases, functional metabolic disorders, musculoskeletal disorders—which make a definitive fibromyalgia diagnosis difficult), and lack of exercise due to fatigue. Standard treatments like massage therapy, prescription medications, dieting, and exercise may not be enough for many fibromites. The reality is, because the condition is not well understood, there is conflicting information on how best to treat it.

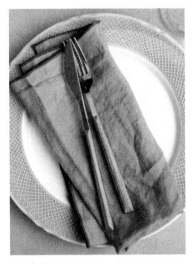

Using my knowledge as a registered dietitian nutritionist and certified LEAP (lifestyle eating and performance) therapist to help fibromites, I have seen firsthand the healing power of specific foods and lifestyle changes. Food sensitivities, inflammation, hormone imbalances, and weight issues can all be mitigated with the right nutrition, and nearly all affected report improved symptoms in a matter of days to weeks.

Fibromyalgia Freedom! outlines exactly how to optimize your health by eating the right foods, using movement, and changing your mind-set. If you feel lost and frustrated with conventional treatment methods or want a natural way to improve your pain and fatigue, this book will help you. You can change your life by taking charge of one of the most important underlying factors that can contribute to pain, fatigue, and brain fog: food.

This book provides a list of foods to consume and enjoy often and advises which foods to eliminate from your diet. The book's 28-day meal plan and 116 delicious recipes were developed to help you move closer to a pain-free life, take charge of your pain, lessen your fatigue, and improve your overall health.

Get ready—you're taking a major step to maximize your life through improving your health. Though your goal may be to manage fibromyalgia, you will see your mind and body heal in the process.

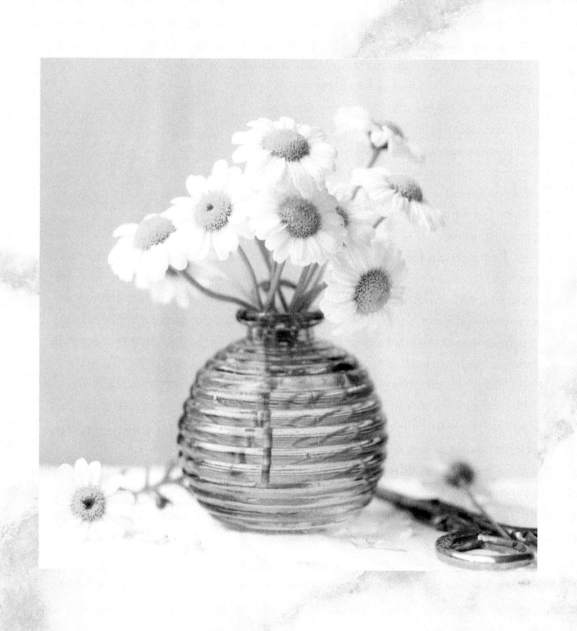

PART I

BREAK UP WITH PAIN

Fibromyalgia can be a puzzling condition. Pain, fatigue, and brain fog have taken over, and you've forgotten what it's like to feel well. The first thing to do in managing your fibromyalgia is to understand the power of food. Because food is information for your cells, it is your most powerful ally in the fight against fibromyalgia. In this part, I explain the fibromyalgia diagnosis, the connection between the nervous system and gastrointestinal systems, hormones and neurotransmitters, and the important role food plays.

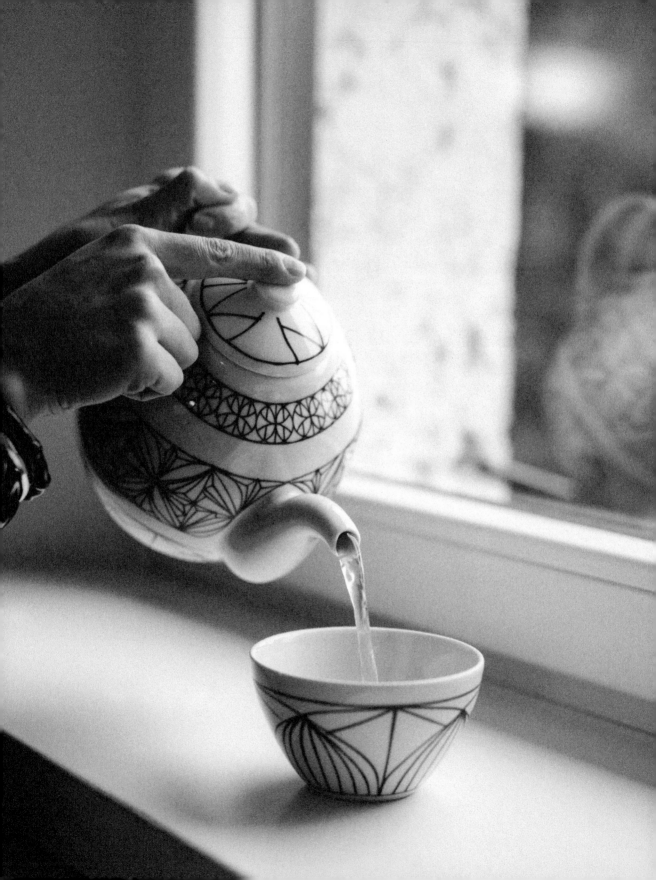

1
understanding fibromyalgia

If you're like me, you've done plenty of research about fibromyalgia. If that's the case, much of what you read in this chapter may be familiar to you. If you've been diagnosed recently, the contents will better familiarize you with fibromyalgia. (If you'd like to learn more, check out the Resources section, page 219, for a list of useful organizations and websites.)

Whenever you consider making changes to your nutrition regimen, consult your health care provider first. The information contained in this book is a great resource, but it is not a substitute for the advice of your health care practitioner.

About Fibromyalgia

Fibromyalgia is a syndrome—a group of symptoms that consistently occur together. A syndrome is like a recipe: Cooks must combine the right ingredients to produce the final dish. With fibromyalgia as the final dish, the gastrointestinal (GI) tract and the immune system are the cooks dispensing the ingredients, which, in this case, are genes, stress, and widespread pain with tender points, fatigue, foggy brain, sleep disturbances, and irritable bowel syndrome.

The GI tract is an incredibly complex system. You may not realize it, but almost all of your nervous system and immune system are located inside your gut (or digestive tract). The digestive tract is also home to trillions of bacteria that communicate with your brain and immune system. If you've ever had a gut feeling, there's a scientific explanation for that. The gut is often called "the second brain." It consists of millions of neurons that make up the enteric nervous system, hormones, and neurotransmitters, which all communicate with the brain through the vagus nerve (which passes through the neck and chest to the abdomen and has pathways throughout the body). This is called the gut-brain axis.

The tissue inside the GI tract is vulnerable because it is exposed to all the contents that pass through it. Suboptimal foods and stress damage this sensitive tissue and the bacteria in the digestive tract. It is important to keep this tissue healthy because, if damaged, the neurotransmitters and hormones made inside the gut—such as serotonin, the feel-good hormone produced in response to eating—will not be produced. It is no coincidence that eating can boost your mood.

In addition to neurons and bacteria, the GI tract is lined with immune cells. These immune cells communicate with food, bacteria, and the brain. If your immune cells sense a threat, like a processed food or unknown chemical, they may react by setting off an inflammatory response. Inflammatory proteins from the immune cells may damage the tissue of the GI tract. When this occurs, the gut's walls open and food, bacteria, and inflammatory proteins make their way into the bloodstream, brain, muscles, and joints. This phenomenon, known as intestinal permeability, contributes to many of your fibromyalgia symptoms.

What Causes Fibromyalgia?

To date, there is no known cause of fibromyalgia, but there are many theories researchers are studying. Brain chemistry, genetics, hormonal imbalances, and stress seem to be the biggest contributors to the development of fibromyalgia. Some experts believe the pain-processing pathways of the central nervous system have somehow become vulnerable and oversensitized.

Brain Chemistry

Brain chemistry is the sum of all the chemical messaging that takes place in the brain. Pain tolerance, movement, mood, thinking, organ function, circadian rhythm, and digestion are dictated by brain chemistry. Neurotransmitters are the proteins that act as the chemical messengers. The amount and type of neurotransmitters produced are in constant flux based on feedback from inside and outside the body, as each messenger has a specific role.

Two of the most important neurotransmitters are serotonin and substance P. Serotonin, a master neurotransmitter, sends signals that determine pain, mood, sexual desire, appetite, sleep, and even social behavior. In addition, it is a messenger that provides signals to almost every system in the body—from the cardiovascular system to the endocrine system. If any of these systems is not working properly, serotonin signaling is altered. Substance P is found in your spinal fluid. It helps communicate sensations of pain to your brain and body. Fibromyalgia patients have low levels of serotonin and high levels of substance P in their spinal fluid. This causes enhanced perceptions of pain, making normal triggers seem very painful.

Genetics

Almost every disorder, including fibromyalgia, can be traced to family history and genes. Most people with fibromyalgia have a family member who also has the disorder. It is important to note that genes do not determine which diseases or disorders you will have, but the combination of genetics and lifestyle factors do. Genes are like switches that can be turned on or off based on the information they're given.

Hormonal Imbalance

Haywire hormones may also be a contributing factor to fibromyalgia. Hormones are like a symphony and must work together in harmony. If one hormone's level is too high or too low, if it cannot get to its destination, or cannot be used by the cells, then all other hormones are affected. Insulin, estrogen, and progesterone levels have all been shown to have profound effects on the nervous system and pain. Insulin levels are commonly higher in fibromites, and low levels of progesterone with high levels of estrogen are common in women with fibromyalgia.

FIBROMYALGIA ACROSS GENDER LINES

It is no secret that women are sensitive to cyclical hormone changes from everything to the monthly menstrual cycle to pregnancy and lactation and, finally, menopause. Nine out of ten people diagnosed with fibromyalgia are women; no one knows exactly why, but it may be due to the complexity of women's hormones and possible underdiagnosis or underreporting in men. Hormone levels have been correlated with pain levels in lactation, menstruation, pregnancy, and menopause.

Although fibromyalgia is commonly thought of as a woman's condition, one in nine cases is a man. Men may not receive the same fibromyalgia treatment or proper diagnosis that women receive, however. It is estimated that the number of men suffering from fibromyalgia could, in fact, be closer to 30 percent. Interestingly, the experience of men with the illness is very different from that of its female sufferers. Overall, men report milder and more acute symptoms than women. They also tend to have less fatigue, tender points, stiffness, and irritable bowel syndrome.

Stress Response

Research shows that stress contributes to pain signaling in fibromites. The body can perceive almost anything as a threat—too much exercise, violence, abuse, processed foods, traffic, or even bad weather. One of the body's responses to stress is pain. If you have chronic stress, the fight-or-flight response, or sympathetic nervous system, is constantly activated. When this part of the nervous system is dominant, you're more likely to experience illnesses and pain. Thankfully, stress can be modified in many ways, including cognitive behavioral therapy, a healthy diet, positive thinking, mindfulness, and exercise.

Signs and Symptoms

Although not everyone has the same experience with fibromyalgia, there are common signs and symptoms. Most fibromites experience widespread chronic pain, chronic fatigue, and brain fog (fibro fog). Many also report irritable bowel syndrome, sleep disorders, headaches, and mood disorders such as anxiety and depression.

Chronic Pain

Chronic pain is the hallmark of fibromyalgia syndrome. There is also a spectrum in the severity of symptoms—for some, just wearing a T-shirt can be painful (allodynia). Others experience widespread pain and dull body aches with or without joint pain.

The good news is that food can help decrease pain sensations. Natural foods have pain-relieving and anti-inflammatory properties and can help with serotonin production. Ginger, extra-virgin olive oil, cruciferous vegetables, meats, and leafy greens contain anti-inflammatory and pain-relieving chemicals. Some of these chemicals are even used to create medications, such as ibuprofen. One can also eat foods that help the body make serotonin, such as turkey, beef, eggs, cheese, chickpeas, sweet potatoes, dark chocolate, and leafy greens.

Chronic Fatigue

Most fibromyalgia sufferers claim they could sleep for days straight and still feel unrested. Chronic fatigue is often caused by disruptions in the natural circadian rhythm. The circadian rhythm is a 24-hour cycle in living things that is modulated by external cues such as food, sunlight, and temperature. Reestablishing the natural circadian rhythm through diet and lifestyle is a powerful way to fight chronic fatigue.

Meal timing, food type, and amounts are key factors in improving circadian rhythm. Eating three meals a day at the same times and avoiding snacking give your GI tract a chance to complete its natural cycle by allowing the migrating motor complex (MMC) to occur in its entirety. The MMC is a "housekeeper" pattern of activity in the GI tract's smooth muscle that sweeps leftover undigested material through the digestive tube and out of the body. The best way to assist the MMC in its completion is to allow longer periods of time between meals—four to five hours is ideal, with nothing to eat or drink except for water. During this time, hormones, neurotransmitters, and immune cells in the GI tract are reset and the body can move waste material out without interruption. Eating sooner immediately stops the MMC in its tracks, contributing to chronic fatigue symptoms.

The type of food you choose for your meals is also very important for circadian rhythm function. Always choose real, whole foods. For each meal, choose a leafy green vegetable, a healthy protein, and a healthy fat. Because the normal circadian rhythm demonstrates a higher serotonin level in the evening hours, add carbohydrates such as a sweet potato, yam, squash, or dark chocolate at dinnertime to help with serotonin production.

Determine the amount you eat by the time of day. Try to eat a medium breakfast, a large lunch, and a medium dinner. Being too full or too hungry at bedtime can disrupt your sleep. Try to give your body a break from food by eating no later than two hours before bed each night.

"Fibro Fog"

Searching for words, short-term memory loss, and feeling like you've taken too much cold/sinus medication are symptoms of fibro fog, also known as cognitive dysfunction or impaired cognition.

Fibro fog is most likely caused by two things: inflammation and oxidative stress. Inflammation is the body's natural response to injury. It is good in the short term, but can damage tissues and zap energy if it goes on for too long. Oxidative stress is an imbalance in the body between free radicals—molecules that have an extra electron, which makes them dangerous and unstable to the body—and the body's natural defense, antioxidants.

When the hypothalamus in the brain senses inflammation or oxidative stress, it responds by shutting down the pathways we need to think clearly. Anything that contributes to oxidative stress or inflammation, such as processed foods, food sensitivities, over exercising, sleep deprivation, disrupted circadian rhythm, and emotional stress, will make brain fog worse.

The good news is, you can buffer inflammation and oxidative stress with the right foods. Vegetables, healthy fats, protein, and fermented foods at each meal are the best defense against fibro fog. Vegetables such as broccoli, asparagus, lettuce, garlic, onions, and kale are loaded with antioxidants that stabilize free radicals. They also provide vitamins and minerals that contribute to the structure and energy-producing functions of cells. Healthy fats such as omega-3s from fish also act as antioxidants and stabilize cell membranes. Animal protein provides all the amino acid building blocks needed to keep tissues healthy and for repair where needed. Fermented foods provide healthy bacteria (probiotics), which buffer inflammation and communicate with the brain, letting it know the environment is safe.

SLEEP BETTER, FEEL BETTER

Getting good sleep is easier said than done when you're struggling with fibromyalgia. Here are a few tips for improving your sleep habits.

- Eat at the same time every day.
- Get some natural sunlight every day, preferably at noon to assure proper hormone production and circadian rhythm function.
- Move as much as you can during the day, and do calming exercises like Pilates, yoga, or light walking in the evening.
- Avoid alcohol and caffeine, as both have direct effects on the nervous system and are known to disrupt circadian rhythms.
- Eat real food and avoid processed foods such as crackers, cookies, cakes, chips, candies, and sodas. There are more than 10,000 legal food additives in the United States contained in these foods, and most negatively affect the nervous system and GI tract, and contribute to inflammation.
- Stop eating two hours before bed to give your body a chance to digest and rest.
- If you're really hungry at bedtime, you may not be able to sleep. Eating a small healthy snack of cheese, peanut butter, or almond butter before bedtime will not adversely affect your sleep.
- Include serotonin-stimulating foods at dinnertime. Almond butter, meats, sweet potatoes, chickpeas, yams, and squash are great options.
- Eliminate all sources of light in your bedroom. Even tiny on/off switches on electronics produce enough light to disrupt your sleep.
- Avoid screen time from electronic devices, like television, computers, and smartphones, at least one hour before bedtime. Blue light from screens can trick the body into thinking it is daytime. If you cannot avoid screen time before bed, consider using amber glasses to block the blue light and turn the brightness/light intensity down on your devices.

Food Fight

Food is the most powerful weapon in your fight against fibromyalgia.

Because you've tried so many things already, you may be skeptical and confused about how changing your diet, yet again, will actually work. The best plan for managing fibromyalgia includes one that teases out the best combination of foods and very specific nutrients. It must also suit your individual set of genes, preferences, and lifestyle.

The diet plan offered in this book is physiologic, meaning natural, and will contribute to your overall health and the optimal function of the nervous system, hormones, and all organs of the body. Healthy bodies have less pain. The guidelines here are a good starting place, and guided trial and error will help determine what foods suit you best.

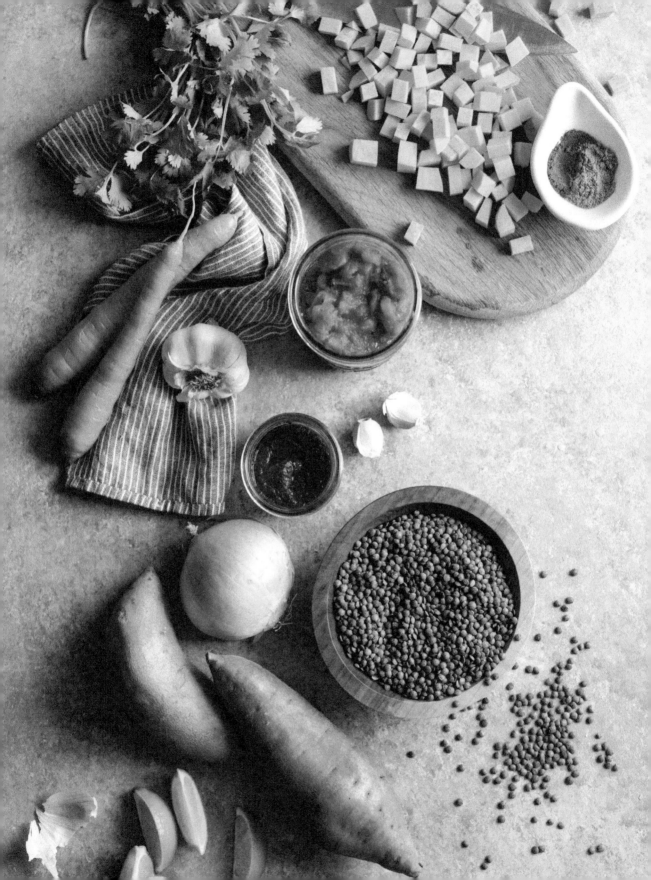

2
food and movement

You've probably heard the saying, "you are what you eat," and it's true—but only to a point. More accurately, you are what your body makes out of what you eat. Because the body is one giant feedback loop, the food you eat has a direct effect on your hormones, immune system, gastrointestinal tract, and the sensitivity of your nervous system. Certain chemicals in the foods you eat may trigger the release of neurotransmitters that increase this sensitivity. On the other hand, eating certain foods can protect and fuel all the body's systems and, most important for fibromyalgia sufferers, the nervous system. This chapter covers the dos and don'ts of the fibromyalgia diet, and looks at how exercise and types of exercises alleviate fibromyalgia symptoms.

Eating Clean and the Fibromyalgia Diet

The fibromyalgia diet is designed to bring you back to your innate physiologic roots to minimize the effects of the syndrome. As you start eating based on your body's natural design, the healing process can begin.

Let's begin by drilling down to the type of foods permitted on the fibromyalgia diet and those to avoid.

Foods to Enjoy

The following foods are the building blocks of the fibromyalgia diet. Having these foods in your kitchen is one of the best weapons you have for pain management.

- Almond butter
- Dark chocolate (more than 85 percent cocoa)
- Dark leafy green vegetables
- Extra-virgin olive oil
- Fermented foods (kimchi, sauerkraut, full-fat yogurt)
- Full-fat dairy (after the 30-day elimination, if no symptoms reoccur when reintroduced)
- Grass-fed meats
- Small fish (sardines, anchovies)
- Sweet potatoes
- Tulsi tea

Foods to Avoid

Eliminating the following foods from your diet helps manage the effects of fibromyalgia. Avoid temptation by taking the time to remove anything on this list from your kitchen. If some foods on this list are typically in your diet, it may be a bit difficult to do without them, but you'll be glad you ditched them when your symptoms begin to abate.

- Alcohol
- Artificial sweeteners (except xylitol)
- Fruit juice
- Grains
- Hydrogenated oils
- Large fish
- Legumes
- Processed foods
- Soda
- Sugar

Eat Your Colors

An easy way to determine whether you're eating healthy is to pay attention to the colors of your foods. If you are eating a variety of colorful vegetables every day, not only are you getting a lot of antioxidants, but you are avoiding toxins as well. The combination of colors from vegetables and some fruit includes nature's best medicine for fighting disease and supporting optimal health.

Leafy greens should be the cornerstone of every meal. Chlorophyll, the green pigment in plants, helps the liver remove harmful compounds from your body. Some experts believe that supporting detoxification can help treat chronic pain.

In addition to leafy greens, cruciferous vegetables, such as broccoli and cabbage, detoxify chemicals before they do damage to the body. Lutein, found in foods such as avocado, spinach, and leafy greens, can assist with normal circadian rhythm.

Blueberries have the highest antioxidant activity of all foods. This is due to a natural chemical called anthocyanin, which makes them blue. Anthocyanins support the cardiovascular system, blood pressure, and healthy clot formation to ensure nutrients can be delivered to all the tissues in the body, including your nervous system. The best way to incorporate anthocyanins in your diet is to eat blue, purple, and pink-colored vegetables such as beets, eggplant, cabbage, onions, and blackberries.

Many people with fibromyalgia avoid nightshade vegetables as they contain alkaloids, which may contribute to inflammation in sensitive individuals. If you are not sensitive to nightshades, eating red vegetables like tomatoes and peppers can be very beneficial. Lycopene, the pigment that makes these foods red, is a powerful anti-inflammatory compound linked to decreased risks of heart disease and cancer. Red vegetables also contain tannins, which prevent harmful bacteria from attaching to cells.

Orange foods, like sweet potatoes, pumpkins, squash, peppers, and carrots, contain beta-carotene (vitamin A precursor) and vitamin C. These foods support immune function, vision, and glucose metabolism. Maximizing these systems will contribute to good pain management.

While color should guide the vegetable choices you make, interestingly, the largest class of plant chemicals are the flavonoids, and most are colorless. Flavonoids are powerful antioxidants, because they assist the body in buffering free radicals. Spinach, onions, broccoli, lettuce, beets, peppers, Brussels sprouts, and dark chocolate contain high amounts of flavanoids.

When choosing your vegetables and fruits (and protein), try to purchase organic produce and animal products. Though there is no guarantee organic produce is free of chemical contamination, the pesticide and herbicide load you get from eating organic produce is less than it is with mass-produced, commercially grown fruits and vegetables. Animals that graze, not eating grain-based feed, have fat and muscle tissue with higher amounts of omega-3 fats, vitamins, and minerals. These animals have tissue and milk that are less inflammatory to a fibromite than conventionally raised livestock and poultry. Grass-fed animals move more, making

MEDICATIONS, VITAMINS, AND MINERALS

Medication prescribed to fibromites is often meant to ease pain. While we're not suggesting you give up your medications, here's a little info on what each commonly prescribed medications does and which foods can produce the same effects. The table also includes vitamins and minerals that help fight fibromyalgia symptoms.

MEDICATION/VITAMIN/MINERAL/FOOD COMPONENT	FOOD/FOOD COMPONENT
ACETAMINOPHEN Pain-reliever that blocks opioid receptors to reduce pain. Easy to find over the counter.	Cherries (anthocyanins), dark chocolate (epicatechins)
MS CONTIN A common pain-reliever given to fibro patients by prescription only.	Cheese (casomorphins), yogurt (acidophilus)
NAPROXEN SODIUM Blocks prostaglandins—hormones involved in pain and inflammation	Anchovies/sardines (omega-3 fatty acids), blueberries (anthocyanins)
NALTREXONE An opiate blocker generally taken at bedtime. It has anti-inflammatory effects.	Coconut oil (lauric acid), curcumin/turmeric, sauerkraut (probiotic bacteria)
SERTRALINE This SSRI (selective serotonin reuptake inhibitor) helps improve mood by increasing serotonin levels in the brain.	Sweet potatoes (serotonin)
PREGABALIN Works to calm the nervous system and, therefore, useful in treating nerve and muscle pain. It is also effective for treating seizures.	Brazil nuts, leafy green vegetables (magnesium)
MAGNESIUM Needed for optimal sleep, brain function, and calming the nervous system.	Leafy greens

MEDICATION/VITAMIN/MINERAL/FOOD COMPONENT	FOOD/FOOD COMPONENT
SULFUR Known as the healing mineral. Sulfur deficiency is associated with pain and inflammation of various muscle and skeletal disorders.	Asparagus, Brussels sprouts, garlic, onions
B-VITAMINS Vitamins B1, B6, and B12 provide relief by targeting pathways associated with central neural pain processing.	Leafy greens, meats
VITAMIN D Counteracts inflammation; vitamin D deficiency has been linked to fibromyalgia and chronic widespread pain.	Dairy, sunlight
VITAMIN C Important due to its antioxidant function. It can help fight the free radicals that exacerbate pain hypersensitivity.	Peppers, tomatoes
SALT Provides the mineral sodium. Sodium helps maintain fluid balance, hydration, and aids in nerve signal transmission.	Chicken broth, Himalayan salt, table salt
ADAPTOGENS Herbs that help with symptoms of fibromyalgia by increasing the body's ability to resist stress and balance hormones.	Tea: Ashwagandha, holy basil/Tulsi, Rhodiola rosea
OMEGA-3 FATTY ACIDS Omega-3s have potent anti-inflammatory and immune-modulating properties.	Fish
ACIDOPHILUS PROBIOTIC BACTERIA Probiotics increase the expression of opioid receptors in intestines and have morphine-like effects.	Full-fat yogurt, sauerkraut
EPICATECHINS These act on opioid receptors, so help decrease pain sensations.	Dark chocolate
CASOMORPHIN AND MENTHOL Both help block pain at opioid receptors.	Cheese, mint
ANTHOCYANINS Pain relieving. They also have anti-inflammatory effects.	Blueberries, cherries, dark purple and red fruits and vegetables
HERBS Some herbs potent anti-inflammatory, pain-relieving, and immune-modulating effects.	Curcumin/turmeric

muscle tissue healthier. They also avoid aflatoxins—chemicals produced by a fungus that grows on grains and animal feed that are poisonous to human cells—often present in conventional feed.

Get Moving

Humans were designed to move, so adding movement to your lifestyle will only make you feel better and contribute to your health. As a lifelong athlete I love exercise, but realize this is not the case for everyone. If you're fighting brain fog, anxiety, fatigue, and other fibro symptoms, the last thing you have the energy for is exercise. But making the Herculean effort to get up and move is well worth the struggle because movement is a powerful tool in your fibro toolbox. A good rule of thumb: Only do exercise you enjoy. Here are five reasons even gentle exercise can ease fibro symptoms.

Fights Brain Fog

Impaired cognition, or brain fog, is one of the most frustrating symptoms experienced by fibromyalgia sufferers. One exercise that counteracts brain fog is rebounding (see page 20). It helps with lymphatic drainage, which clears brain fog. Plus, jumping on a trampoline is just plain fun. Studies have shown that exercise improves several aspects of cognition and has been correlated with memory improvement. The mechanism behind these effects may be due to dopamine. Interestingly, dopamine production increases in response to exercise.

Decreases Anxiety

Fear, worry, and hypervigilance go hand in hand with an oversensitive nervous system, so it comes as no surprise that most people with fibromyalgia suffer from anxiety. Strength training and high-intensity interval training have both been shown to reduce anxiety. Most of my patients almost always report feeling relieved of worry after a good sweat session.

Counteracts Chronic Fatigue

About one-fourth of Americans experience chronic fatigue. Fatigue is a catch-22 because you need exercise to improve energy, but if you're tired, you probably don't want to work out. Study after study has shown exercise to be clinically beneficial, and it can even be more beneficial than drug or cognitive behavioral interventions (O'Connor, Herring, and Caravalho). Lifting weights or strength training provides the largest benefit for counteracting chronic fatigue.

Improves Sleep

Never underestimate the effect of sleep—or lack thereof—on your health and well-being. Consistent sleep deprivation (fewer than six hours a night) is associated with cognitive impairment, mental illness, obesity, daytime sleepiness, and a diminished quality of life (O'Connor, Herring, and Caravalho). Thankfully, there's a way to improve sleep: exercise. Physically active people demonstrate better sleep patterns and a lower risk of sleep apnea. Sleep apnea is associated with decreased pain threshold. Studies have shown the benefit of exercise in depressed and sleep-deprived subjects. People who added regular resistance training to their lifestyle had improved sleep by 30 percent after 8 to 10 weeks.

Better Mental Health

Exercise triggers a network of neurophysiological adaptations that affect mental and emotional function. Resistance training improves central nervous system function, which has positive effects on mental health through several mechanisms. Exercise helps your body make new nerve cells—neurotransmitters for more efficient oxygen and nutrient delivery to tissues—for a better overall feeling.

SETS AND REPS

The amount of time, intensity, and type of exercise you do depends on your baseline—your starting point. If you are sedentary, start with walking: 30 minutes every day, or 5,000 to 10,000 steps per day. I measure my steps using a Fitbit watch.

If you already walk regularly, add some strength training three to four times per week for 30 minutes at a time, and maybe even some interval training for 10 minutes once or twice per week.

If you are struggling and don't know where to start, consider hiring a professional personal trainer to get you going.

Rebounding. If you don't like exercise or are not sure where to start, consider jumping on an adult mini trampoline. You can purchase one almost anywhere for less than $50. Jumping on a trampoline is one of best forms of exercise. It is fun, easy on the joints, and, due to negative G-forces, it helps with lymphatic drainage. All these properties are important for pain management. Put on your favorite music and dance while you jump. You don't need to have a specific routine—just enjoy jumping for 15 to 20 minutes every other day.

Kettlebells. Kettlebells are cannonball-shaped weights with handles. Add exercises using them to your routine if you want a stronger, tighter core without spending much time on it. Kettlebells are great because they are easy to work with and promote functional, real-world movement in the same way everyday activities do, like carrying a toddler, hoisting a gallon of milk, or lifting a heavy grocery bag. Kettlebell swings get your heart rate up and help strengthen your muscles all in one movement. A strong core is key to pain management and overall healthy neuromuscular function. Swinging a kettlebell is also a lot of fun and provides stress relief. There are many good YouTube and Web tutorials on how to use a kettlebell. My favorite is a workout by Jillian Michaels called "Shred-It with Weights."

Posture Work. Posture work includes Pilates, yoga, and PostureFit. They are all fun and simple exercises you can add to your at-home routine. If you've had a rough day and are looking for a lower level of intensity, posture work is a good choice. These exercises are somewhat demanding, but not the kind of workout that always works up a sweat. The main concept is about concentration and breathing, and paying close attention to how your muscles feel during each exercise. These mainly target your core, legs, glutes, and back and boost flexibility to help with joint mobility. There are many good websites and YouTube videos available for posture work. My favorites are Jennifer Kries, PostureFit Bar/System, and Tara Stiles. Aim for 15 minutes every other day. Avoid any exercises that cause pain.

Swimming. The natural pressure of water against your body (hydrostatic pressure) is very therapeutic. Immersion in water also creates buoyancy, so it does not put strain on your joints. Pick any stroke and swim for 30 minutes a couple times a week. If you like classes, join a water aerobics class at your local pool. Even if you're not a great swimmer, any movement you do in the water will help strengthen your muscles and heart, contribute to a higher metabolic rate, and provide pain relief.

Walking Intervals. Find a nice place outside to enjoy nature and do some brisk walking. Walking intervals are a great way to boost your metabolism and endorphins. Find a short, steep hill, and walk up as quickly as you can and catch your breath on the way down. For longer hills, time a fast interval of about 60 seconds followed by 60 seconds to catch your breath. Repeat 10 times and then cool down while walking down the hill. Breathe deeply and fill your lungs with air. Intervals are good for every system in the body and will quickly get you into great shape. Enjoy these walking intervals every day, if you like—30 minutes is all you need to benefit.

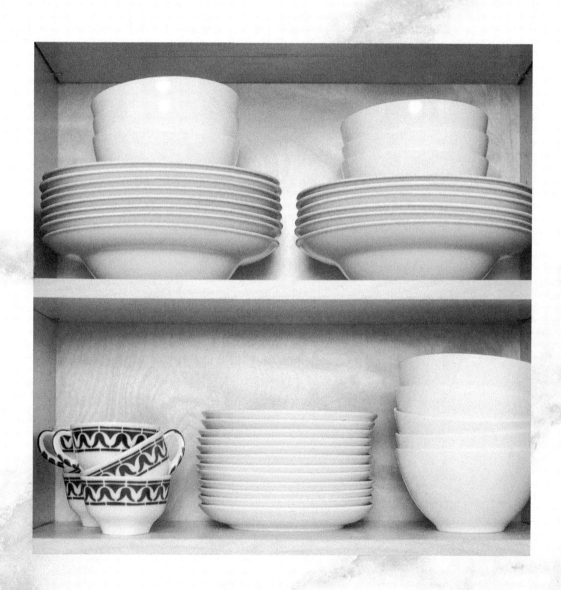

PART 2

THE PLAN

In this part, we'll focus on the plan, creating the foundation for healthy habits in 28 days. Here, you'll find actionable steps to put your knowledge into practice with an easy-to-follow meal plan and delectable recipes crafted for your specific needs. You should see tangible improvement in symptoms after completing the meal plan, but it is unlikely you will be completely pain free in that short time. Continued experimentation with the recipes in this book will take the guesswork out of what to eat in your daily life.

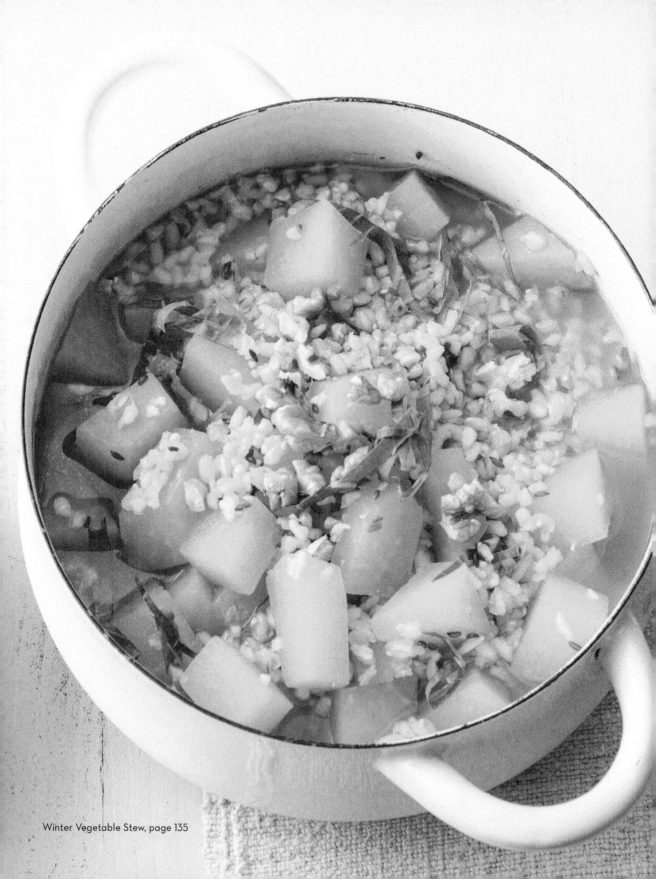

Winter Vegetable Stew, page 135

3

four weeks to fibro freedom!

While you can try sticking to the diet on your own, it usually helps to have a meal plan with shopping lists and recipes planned for you, just to start. That's where this meal plan comes in. Once you feel on firm footing with the diet and have at least one month under your belt following the meal plan, you'll have the confidence to step outside of this book to find your own fibro-friendly recipes, while still having the recipes here to fall back on.

28-Day Meal Plan

The fibro diet excludes foods that exacerbate pain and includes foods that are neutral or decrease symptoms of the syndrome. To review the fibromyalgia diet—what foods can you include? What foods should you exclude?—go back to Eating Clean and the Fibromyalgia Diet on page 13 in chapter 2.

This 28-Day Meal Plan makes getting and staying on the fibro diet easy—your meals are planned, all the shopping lists are made, all the portions are measured.

Before jumping into eliminating foods and diving into the fibro diet (using the meal plan), you want to see where you are right now. That means taking a baseline of all your fibro symptoms. To start, record all your symptoms in detail for at least two weeks before starting the 28-Day Meal Plan, so you have a baseline from which to compare. Write down what you eat, when you eat it, immediate responses, and any symptoms that worsen or change after a meal. Also, compile a list of chronic symptoms. Use the Symptom Log (page 31) and the Food and Symptom Journal (page 33) to record your baseline. You may start to see patterns with respect to food intake and how you feel, which will start to explain how diet and your condition are linked.

Use this two-week baseline-recording period to clean out your pantry and refrigerator slowly of foods that are not in the fibro diet. While the idea is to see how you function on your regular diet, if you use up something in the course of the two weeks that is not on the fibro diet, such as a bag of refined sugar, don't go out and purchase a new one.

After creating a comprehensive baseline, it's time to jump into the fibro diet and get rid of those foods that cause pain and all the other symptoms you're trying to decrease or eliminate. Faithfully following the meal plan with no cheating is your best shot at keeping the elimination period short.

There are very few people, if any, who can start a new diet plan, especially one focused on elimination, and not have a few setbacks. Commit to the fibro diet for 28 days to track the changes in your body. If you slip up and eat something not on the plan, just move on and make a note of the circumstances, such as your emotional feelings and, of course, any physical reactions to the food.

Be prepared for the possibility that you might not see any improvement right away. Your progress will depend on your baseline condition and how strictly you follow the plan. Do not give up if you do not experience miracle improvements from changing your diet. Some people notice improvement in their symptoms right away, and others experience a more gradual change. Even if you feel much better, it's still important to continue the diet until all your symptoms subside completely, then follow the reintroduction process. If you do not see diminished symptoms, consult your doctor for strategies.

After successfully following the meal plan, it's time to try reintroducing some of the eliminated foods back into your diet to see which ones you can keep in your diet and which ones you need to stay away from long term.

The following sections cover each step of elimination, reintroduction, and tracking symptoms (including charts showing exactly how to track progress and symptoms successfully), helping you take control of your nutrition to manage your fibromyalgia.

Deconstruct and Reconstruct

You're probably excited to jump right into this diet so you can see some improvement in your fibromyalgia symptoms. But first, it is a good idea to get an inventory of your health before you start the meal plans. This baseline of symptoms, emotions, and reactions is valuable so you can refer to them during the four-week diet plan (see pages 30–33 for step-by-step instructions on how to record your baseline of symptoms).

The fibromyalgia diet, explained in chapter 2, is an elimination diet designed to remove any foods that are known allergens or cause negative reactions, so you'll notice many popular ingredients missing from the recipes, such as gluten, pseudo grains (quinoa, teff, buckwheat, wild rice, amaranth, etc.), legumes, sugar, and most fruit. This list is not comprehensive, so avoid any other foods—such as nightshades (tomatoes, peppers, eggplants, and others) or nuts (any nut you're allergic to)—that you know increase your symptoms.

Elimination diets are designed to remove all foods that cause adverse reactions from your meals so your body has an opportunity to heal. The length of time that you follow the elimination diet will depend on your baseline condition and the extent of damage present in your body. The minimum time frame is four weeks and there is no maximum time frame (though if you see no improvement, or very little, after four weeks and have been following the fibro diet diligently with no lapses, have a discussion your medical practitioner to pinpoint what might be stalling your progress). Continue to follow the plan until your symptoms are no longer evident or have improved considerably.

The best way to start an elimination diet is to clear out your refrigerator and pantry of excluded foods, go shopping, and start eating fibromyalgia-friendly meals immediately. While you can transition more slowly, your health will improve more quickly with this cold-turkey strategy. The elimination diet does not officially start until you exclude all restricted foods.

The first few days on any new plan are difficult, even if you are optimistic about changing your diet. Don't worry, there are lots of delicious recipes in this book so you will not feel deprived, and remember: An elimination diet is *temporary*. Your diet journey will be unique to you, as will your body's reaction to the elimination phase. Though it's hard to predict how long the elimination portion of the diet will last, continue to track your physical reactions to pinpoint when you can start reintroducing foods. Food reintroduction can start when symptoms subside. The meal plans will show what you eat, so all you need to do is record when you eat, immediate responses (if there are any), and any symptoms that worsen or change after a meal. Remember, if you see no changes in symptoms in four weeks, talk to your doctor.

Food Reintroduction Plan and Symptom Trackers

The reintroduction process can be very exciting because you add different foods back into your diet. The most important thing to remember in this phase is not to rush the process; following the guidelines ensures a better chance for success. Follow the meal plan or, at a minimum, the fibromyalgia diet, for 30 days with no cheating as well as the lifestyle recommendations, such as managing sleep and stress, and exercise goals. Do not attempt to reintroduce foods until your symptoms improve, because you do not want to sabotage your progress.

This reintroduction phase is based on principles of the LEAP protocol, which focuses on *nonreactive foods* (those less likely to cause negative symptoms) rather than reactive foods (those that contribute to inflammation, brain fog, and pain). If you struggle with inflammation, you may experience problems with foods like milk and dairy, eggs, nuts, gluten, seeds, potatoes, nightshades, coffee, and alcohol. Removing these foods from your diet for 30 days allows your immune system to calm and reset itself. After those 30 days, the immune system is less likely to react negatively to common offenders when they are reintroduced into your diet. In other words, the immune system does not remember them, so it does not react in a defensive manner. Of course, it is ideal to have a mediator release blood test (MRT®) performed by your doctor or dietitian to determine your specific food sensitivities. If you do not have access to testing, following the steps outlined here should give you a good idea as to which foods you can reintroduce first, and which you can reintroduce down the road (in two to three months) to calm and reset your immune system.

Be prepared: It may take months to reintroduce some foods successfully back into your daily diet—and some foods may need to be eliminated permanently.

However, knowing which ingredients cause negative reactions in your body is a positive step because you can now control some of your symptoms. It will take time to get through the list of foods you have eliminated, so patience is key. You need to reintroduce ingredients one at a time to see exactly what your reaction is to that food only. Foods to eliminate for 30 days are common offenders, but may be included in the *Fibromyalgia Freedom!* meal plan: alcohol, cheese, coffee, eggs, milk, nightshades, nuts, and seeds.

In the reintroduction phase, you will introduce foods that are less likely to cause reactions first and move on to foods that are more likely to cause a reaction. This order shouldn't leave you with a serious flare-up before you have a few successes. Keep in mind, your food intolerances are unique to you, so there is no way to predict which foods will cause reactions unless you've had a mediator release test. Some foods in the fibromyalgia diet, such as nightshades or full-fat dairy, might be a problem for you, so looking at the symptom tracker is important. You can add those foods to your reintroduction list as needed, placing nightshades such as bell peppers, eggplant, and tomatoes closer to the end of the process.

Here is how reintroduction works:

1. After giving up common offenders for 30 days (see page 28), pick one common offender food (see list on page 30) to reintroduce.
2. Try a small amount of your first common offender food and, over the next three days, closely monitor for symptoms or potential reactions. Look for changes such as the reappearance or increase of mental fog, rashes, joint pain, inflammation, digestive problems, fatigue, and sleep disruption. If you have a reaction at any point in this process, stop eating that challenge food. You can try to reintroduce it after another 30 days.
3. If you have no reaction over the three-day trial period, continue eating the first challenge food in small amounts and introduce a second challenge food at this time. Over the next three days, watch closely for potential reactions as listed in step 2. If adverse symptoms appear, eliminate the common offender and reintroduce it again in 30 days.
4. If you continue to experience no reactions, continue to eat the challenge food(s) in larger amounts. Monitor yourself closely for negative reactions. If you have no reaction after a week, the common offender food is safe to add back to your diet.

5. Continue this process with the list of common offenders, reintroducing a new common offender every three days, until you can eat full portions of your challenge food without any adverse effects. If adverse symptoms appear, eliminate the common offender and reintroduce it in 30 days.

6. Continue with the list until common offenders are reintroduced or saved for later reintroduction.

Keep in mind that there is a dose-response when it comes to food sensitivity. For example, one piece of cheese may not be bothersome, but three or four pieces may cause reactions. It is best to avoid overeating any foods at all times.

Reintroduce these foods one at a time, *in this order*:

- Milk
- Cheese
- Nuts

- Eggs
- Potatoes
- Seeds

- Coffee
- Alcohol
  (after 60 days)

During reintroduction, track what you eat, when you eat it, and your symptoms (if any), so you have a record of your reactions. Write down everything, positive and negative reactions, to get an accurate picture of how the challenge foods affect your body. Keep track of other aspects of your life, too, during this time, such as:

- Any fibromyalgia symptoms and any changes
- Any other changes in your routine
- Digestion

- Emotions
- Energy levels
- Pain and where (rated on a scale of 0 to 10)

- Sleep quality and how you feel when you wake up

Track Your Symptoms

Recording your symptom baseline, weekly progress, and the foods you eat with the correlating reactions in your body is a valuable strategy to regaining control of your health. This type of tracking activity takes less time than you might think, so commit to the process to get the best results for this diet.

SYMPTOM LOG

No symptoms: 0, Mild: 1–3, Moderate: 4–6, Severe: 7–9, Very Severe: 10

SYMPTOMS	MONDAY	TUESDAY	WEDNESDAY	THURSDAY	FRIDAY	SATURDAY	SUNDAY
Abdominal Pain							
Depression							
Dizziness/ Balance							
Fatigue							
Fogginess/ Memory							
Headache							
Joint Pain							
Light Sensitivity							
Lymph Node Tenderness							
Mood Changes							
Pain							
Poor Sleep							
Sore Throat							

WEEKLY SYMPTOM DIARY

Week Starting: _____

	SYMPTOMS A.M.	SYMPTOMS P.M.
MONDAY		
TUESDAY		
WEDNESDAY		
THURSDAY		
FRIDAY		
SATURDAY		
SUNDAY		

FOOD AND SYMPTOM JOURNAL

DATE	TIME	FOOD/BEVERAGE	QUANTITY	SYMPTOMS/SEVERITY	TIME SYMPTOMS STOPPED

EATING MINDFULLY

You probably have heard the word *mindful* in relation to strategies for life changes and becoming more self-aware, but mindful eating may be a new concept. Put simply, when you eat mindfully, you pay attention when you are eating. Consider the opposite of this idea—eating mindlessly—and think back on a moment when you were watching TV and spooning your dinner into your mouth without much attention to what is on your plate or how much you eat.

Mindful eating means paying attention to

- your food choices
- enjoyment and nourishment from those foods
- the way your food looks and smells
- the food's taste and texture
- how you feel during and after the meal
- how full you feel
- why you are eating (hunger or emotional triggers)
- your physical and emotional feelings for the rest of your day

The mindful eating process makes you more aware and appreciative of both your food and how eating is linked to physical and emotional well-being. Eating mindfully also makes you aware of when you reach fullness because you pay attention to your body's cues. Paying attention to your meals relaxes your mind, decreasing your stress levels. Mindful eating is not difficult, but it may take some time to get used to because eating patterns are habits, and breaking existing ones to implement new ones takes time.

Here are some simple steps to get started on mindful eating:

- Eliminate all distractions—that means no books, newspapers, smartphones, tablets, television, etc.
- Eat more slowly; no matter what, don't rush your meals.
- Put your fork or spoon down between bites.
- Chew slowly and thoroughly.
- Take smaller bites and sips.
- Stop eating when you're full.
- Think about why you are eating (hungry, bored, sad, etc.).

Setting Up Your Kitchen

Getting the right foods into your kitchen, getting rid of inflammatory foods, and having equipment that makes your life easy are all small steps you can take to set yourself up for success—and closer to decreasing your fibro symptoms. What do you need in your pantry? As a fibromite, how do you shop for groceries? What equipment is a must? This section answers all your questions.

Pantry Staples

The key to following a diet plan is to stock your kitchen with the ingredients permitted on the diet, so you always have what you need at your fingertips. The following ingredients are the basics required to make the recipes in this cookbook. When following the meal plans, look at the shopping lists and check off the items you already have and make note of any that are getting low.

Lean Grass-Fed or Pasture-Raised Meats and Poultry

- Beef
- Chicken
- Lamb
- Pork
- Turkey
- Venison

Small Wild-Caught Fish and Seafood

- Bass
- Catfish
- Flounder
- Mussels
- Scallops
- Shrimp
- Sole
- Tilapia
- Trout

Dairy and Dairy Substitutes

- Almond milk, unsweetened
- Butter, grass-fed
- Coconut milk, unsweetened
- Cottage cheese and ricotta cheese, full-fat
- Cream cheese
- Eggs
- Heavy (whipping) cream
- Kefir
- Yogurt, plain, full-fat

Freezer

- Berries, frozen
- Edamame
- Vegetables, flash-frozen

Dry Goods and Pantry

- 85 to 90 percent dark chocolate
- Almond flour
- Arrowroot powder
- Baking soda
- Broth, beef, gluten-free, sodium-free
- Broth, chicken, gluten-free, sodium-free
- Broth, vegetable, gluten-free, sodium-free
- Chickpeas
- Cocoa powder, unsweetened
- Coconut aminos
- Coconut cream
- Coconut flour
- Coconut, shredded, unsweetened
- Gelatin
- Ghee
- Oil, coconut
- Oil, olive, extra-virgin
- Oil, sesame
- Olives, Kalamata
- Pumpkin, canned, puréed
- Sauerkraut
- Tomatoes, diced, canned, sodium-free
- Tomatoes, sun-dried
- Tahini
- Vanilla extract, alcohol-free
- Vinegar, apple cider
- Vinegar, balsamic

Nuts and Seeds

- Almond butter
- Almonds
- Cashews
- Flaxseed
- Hazelnuts
- Pecans
- Pistachios
- Pumpkin seeds
- Sesame seeds
- Sunflower seeds
- Walnuts

Sweeteners

- Xylitol

Herbs and Spices

- Basil
- Black pepper, freshly ground
- Chives
- Cilantro
- Cinnamon
- Cloves
- Coriander
- Cumin
- Dill
- Dried chiles
- Garlic
- Ginger
- Himalayan salt or table salt
- Nutmeg
- Oregano
- Parsley
- Rosemary
- Sage
- Tarragon
- Thyme
- Turmeric

Fresh Vegetables

- Artichoke
- Asparagus
- Bell peppers
- Broccoli
- Brussels sprouts
- Butternut squash
- Cabbage
- Carrots
- Cauliflower
- Celery
- Cucumbers
- Fennel
- Garlic
- Jalapeño peppers
- Kale
- Leeks
- Mushrooms
- Onion, red
- Onion, sweet
- Parsnip
- Romaine lettuce
- Scallion
- Spinach
- Sprouts
- Sweet potato
- Swiss chard
- Tomatoes
- Zucchini

Fresh Fruits

- Avocado
- Blueberries
- Coconut
- Grapefruit, ruby red
- Lemon
- Lime
- Orange
- Pomegranate
- Raspberries
- Strawberries

Shopping Guide

The fibromyalgia diet features fresh produce and grass-fed or pasture-raised proteins. These ingredients are typically a bit more expensive than processed foods, but with a little planning, you can eat foods that support good health and stay within your budget. Here are some tips to make the fibromyalgia diet a bit more cost-effective.

Shop seasonal and at farmers' markets: You might not live in an area with farmers' markets or it could be difficult to get to them, but try to do so whenever possible. You can also get seasonal local produce in your grocery store, so take the time to look at the labels on the bins. Seasonal fruit and vegetables, especially locally grown, are less expensive than imported products, taste better, are fresher, and have higher nutritional content. Farmers and vendors want to sell their produce at peak when there is an abundance, and the price reflects this fact. Also, you will not be paying the extra charges associated with shipping the foods across the country if the grower is in your region.

Buy high-quality frozen vegetables and fruit: Although fresh is best, in general, there are times when frozen is just as good. The freezing process for produce has improved such that today, flash-frozen vegetables and fruit lose very little of their nutrients. Frozen vegetables are less expensive than fresh, and you can easily measure just what you need and place the remainder back in the freezer for future use. This cuts down on waste, and unless you are making a salad, frozen products produce great recipe results.

Buy in bulk: Buying food in larger quantities is usually less expensive than smaller packages. Large packages of meat or poultry can be divided up, rewrapped, and frozen for future use. Look for sales—when ground beef is at a stellar price, you can stock up and freeze the excess for when you need it. Purchase shelf-stable items such as oils, dried herbs, and spices in large containers. Just make sure you use them before their expiration date.

Buy bone-in or less expensive cuts of meat: Prime beef cuts have a wonderful reputation, but there is more flavor in the less expensive products like bone-in cuts or ground beef. Also, don't pass up organ meats—they are inexpensive and incredibly nutritious. Liver, heart, and kidneys can be delicious when prepared well, and if you really don't like eating them on their own, try hiding them in casseroles, meatloaf, or meatballs.

Essential Equipment

You probably have most items needed to create the recipes in this book, but some of these tools will help you save time, reduce chopping, and ensure the best results. Here is the essential equipment you might need for recipe preparation:

Baking dishes: Perfect cooking vessels for casseroles, desserts, roasting proteins, and many other culinary applications, get an assortment of sizes from 4-ounce ramekins to larger dishes that hold 4 to 5 quarts and have lids.

Baking sheets: Metal or silicone baking sheets with a minimum 1-inch rim can be used to prepare desserts, fish, meats, vegetables, and make fun foods such as sun-dried tomatoes. If you want professional-grade products, look for three-quarter or two-third sheet pans because a full sheet pan will not fit in most home ovens.

Blender: A handy tool if you do not have a food processor or if you like to make lots of smoothies. Look for a model that crushes ice easily and comes apart for easy cleanup.

Cutting boards: Having cutting boards designated for meats, vegetables, and seafood is crucial for safe food preparation. They come in different sizes, making it easy to have the correct size for your task at hand.

Food processor: You can do all your chopping, grating, slicing, and puréeing with absolutely no effort and in a very short amount of time. Look for a processor with a 10- to 12-cup capacity.

High-quality knives: Professional chefs know a perfectly balanced, finely honed knife is a joy to use and makes any task easier. Head to a kitchen store and hold the knives to determine which is the best length, weight, and shape for your hand. Get a few types including paring, standard chef's, and utility knives.

Measuring cups and spoons: The success of recipes often depends on accurate measurements—especially when baking—so invest in a complete set of wet and dry measuring cups, and measuring spoons ranging from ⅛ teaspoon to 1 tablespoon.

Nonstick cookware: Pots, pans, and skillets are required equipment to prepare recipes, so a selection of different sizes of each will make your life easier. If you want the minimum number required, invest in one large skillet, a larger stockpot for soups, and three saucepans (large, medium, and small).

Peeler and zester: These tools are convenient for preparing root vegetables and zesting citrus fruits. You can also use a peeler to make vegetable noodles.

Stainless steel bowls: Nested bowls never go to waste when you are cooking healthy meals from scratch. Stainless steel is the best material because it is easy to clean and does not stain or rust.

A Note on Slow Cooking

Though not required for the recipes in this book, a slow cooker is a huge time saver. This appliance turns less expensive cuts of meat into tender, flavor-packed meals. Slow cookers usually make large serving amounts, so leftovers are guaranteed and you will not spend as much time in the kitchen.

What to Expect

When embarking on any new food plan, including this one, there are a few things to take into account.

Changing the way you eat can be time-consuming at first. You may have to find a new grocery store or farmers' market, search the aisles for unfamiliar foods, or spend a lot more time in the kitchen. Changing your nutrition habits is not an easy feat, but the long-term benefits are nothing but positive if you stick to the plan. Some short-term effects of changing habits may be difficult to work through, and at first, you may feel overwhelmed. But keep at it—eventually you will get into a routine and enjoy long-term health and wellness.

There is also a social element to making drastic changes to your diet. You may find it difficult to stay on course if surrounded by others eating the standard American diet. Enlist your family, friends, and coworkers to join your healthy lifestyle—they, too, will benefit from eating nutritious meals. There is a lot of truth to the saying, "You are only as healthy as the people around you." Surround yourself with like-minded people. If none in your social circle is inclined to eating healthy, you may find fellow gym members who share your enthusiasm for health, or look to online forums, or join local walking groups.

No matter the social situation, there is always a healthy option. Here are some tips for when you dine out:

- If possible, look at the menu ahead of time and plan what you'll eat before you get to the restaurant.
- Swap fries, potatoes, rice, or pasta for a side salad, and say no to the bread or biscuit basket if it comes around.
- Order your burger without the bun.
- Avoid ketchup and barbecue sauce because they are high in sugar. Salt your food, or add mayo or a little bit of Ranch dressing instead for some extra flavor.
- Order decaf coffee with heavy cream for dessert.
- Ward off peer pressure. If friends or family try to pressure you into eating foods that aren't on the fibro diet, remind them you are making choices to keep your body happy and healthy.

When you begin the fibromyalgia diet, you may have some short-term side effects as your body flushes out highly processed foods and other toxic materials from your system. Some things you may experience are a lack of appetite, muscle cramps, fatigue, or trouble sleeping. This is due to changes in hormones and neuro-transmitters as you withdraw from certain foods. This is normal and, thankfully, not permanent. I experienced leg cramps, headaches, fatigue, and very deep sleep when I transitioned to a high-fat, whole-foods diet. I relied on magnesium supplements and chicken broth, put extra salt on my food, and increased my water consumption to treat the symptoms. Having enough salt in your diet from broth or seasoning is key when you've decreased sugar and insulin levels drop. Lower insulin levels mean lower sodium and water levels in the body. I also decreased my exercise frequency and intensity and got some extra rest. After a couple of weeks, I felt so much better, which made dealing with the short-term discomfort completely worth it.

The long-term benefits of changing how you eat will be a boost in cognition, memory, and mood, fewer aches and less pain, deep sleep, increased energy levels, hunger reduction, reduced insulin levels, and weight loss.

It is also important to note there are two aspects to pain: sensory and emotional. The *sensory* aspect of pain is caused by stimulation of the pain receptors.

The *emotional* aspect is the pleasantness or unpleasantness of the pain. So pain is a subjective feeling that is unique to individuals and situations. Your current physical state, previous experience with pain, and knowledge of the stimulus, can all affect the interpretation of a pain signal. For most people, specific foods can either be a source of great joy or pain. I once had a friend tell me she would never eat broccoli, because her dad used to feed it to her forcefully as a child. This was a source of emotional pain for her, so broccoli is best left off the list for now no matter how healthy it may be. On the other hand, eating chocolate chip cookies all the time because they remind you of your grandma and boost your mood is not the best way to treat your pain and fatigue. Because they are not very rich in nutrients your body needs to recover, those types of food are fine once in a while, but if eaten too often, can do more harm than good. Tending to the emotional aspect of pain in combination with good nutrition can be the biggest contributor to your success in pain management.

Tips and Tricks for Success

It is true that the fibromyalgia diet excludes some foods you probably eat everyday such as bread, fruit, and grains. If this is disheartening, keep in mind that, besides improving your condition, the strictest version of this diet is not meant to be permanent. Don't let any setbacks that crop up during the initial phase, like having a bit of bread, discourage you from your goals. Get back on track and keep going. Here are some tips for success to address some common issues and problems that might occur.

> *Try cooking shortcuts.* The fibromyalgia plan is designed around fresh home-cooked meals, which may be daunting if you have not spent a great deal of time in the kitchen. Fresh ingredients are best, but packaged precut or shredded vegetables, chopped herbs, and good-quality frozen or canned products are perfectly acceptable when you are in pain or fatigued. Using a food processor or mandoline for food preparation can also save time and effort. You can also double a recipe to create leftovers or meals to be frozen for later.

Have a great support team. This is *your* journey, but having supportive people in your life is invaluable. An encouraging hug from a friend or family member when you feel overwhelmed can actually lower stress and cortisol levels in your body. If you do not have a support network, you can certainly find many fabulous online communities or groups in your areas whose members would be delighted to talk you through challenges and share in your successes.

Tackle food cravings. Switching to a strict elimination diet can create food cravings for emotional and physical reasons. If you have a large cup of coffee every morning with a bagel and cream cheese, for example, it will take some time to adjust to your new morning habit. Caffeine is an addictive substance, so you will experience withdrawal symptoms such as headaches. Give the diet at least two weeks for you to get over the initial cravings and understand that foods will seem more desirable because you can't have them. Stay the course and in no time, you will create new habits around foods in this plan.

Minimize stress. Stress can trigger fibromyalgia symptoms, so reducing it can decrease anxiety and depression, and allow you to get better-quality sleep. When the body is stressed it reacts by producing adrenaline, the fight-or-flight response. Ongoing stress in your life means this release of chemicals from the adrenals, as well as other endocrine glands, becomes chronic. The resulting chemical imbalance can create a dysfunction in the autonomic nervous system, leading to increased fibromyalgia symptoms. Managing stress in your life through exercise, meditation, yoga, reading—whatever works for you—will reduce the risk of fibro flares and give the diet plan a better chance to work.

Keep a daily journal. Keeping a written account of your symptoms, events in your life, and emotional health (through your Symptom Logs and Food and Symptom Journal, see pages 31–33) is crucial for understanding the connection among all these factors. Regularly looking back on your logs uncovers patterns that show specific relationships between, for example, a long project at work and muscle pain or fatigue. The logs will also show progressive improvement and which of your actions may have contributed to declining symptoms, such as cutting out gluten or dairy.

Stay hydrated. One universal recommendation in most diets is to drink lots of water, and this holds true for the fibromyalgia plan. Hydrating the cells adequately is not the only reason to drink water; dehydration can also cause fatigue, muscle pain, and poor blood flow, which also affect the oxygenation of muscles. If you do not like water, try coconut water, ginger tea, fresh vegetable juices (such as cucumber), unsweetened almond milk, and herbal teas.

About the Recipes

The recipes in the following chapters use ingredients packed with nutrients and selected specifically for the fibromyalgia diet. Each recipe is labeled with one or more of the following categories to help you pick the dishes that suit your needs.

Brain Booster: This label means the ingredients in the recipe support healthy brain function.

Dairy-Free: These recipes do not contain any milk products.

Gluten-Free: These recipes do not contain any gluten.

Immune Booster: This label means the ingredients in the recipe fight inflammation. These whole foods usually are high in antioxidants and phytonutrients.

Nut-Free: These recipes do not contain any nuts or nut products.

Paleo-Friendly: The ingredients in these recipes conform to the Paleo diet.

Vegetarian: There is no meat, poultry, fish, or seafood ingredients in these recipes. Note that these dishes are not always vegan.

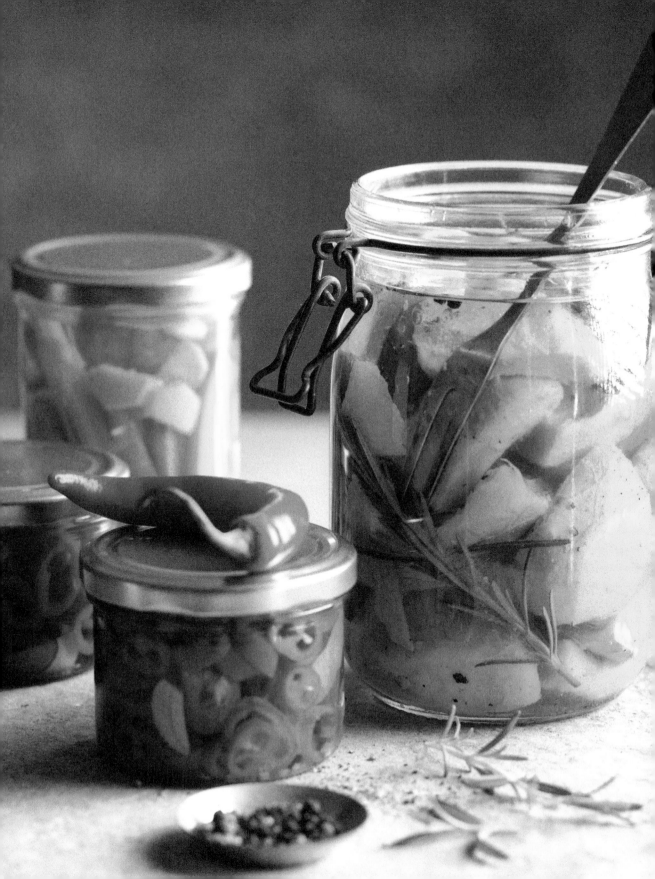

4

meal plans

In this chapter, we dig into the meal plans. It's recommended that you follow them in order, but if brain fog is a larger issue for you than pain management, feel free to start there. Many foods in the fibro diet will address all four areas of concern (pain management, gaining energy, fighting brain fog, and promoting healthy digestion), so don't be surprised to see the same recipes in different sections. This flexibility also makes changing the meal plans possible if you want to double a recipe or try a different one. Just remember to change the shopping lists as well to reflect the different ingredients. The shopping lists probably look long, but in many cases, the pantry items, like extra-virgin olive oil and chicken broth, may already be in your cupboards. There are amounts for needed ingredients on the lists, so take the time to check the pantry, freezer, and refrigerator to see what you already have and check off that item before shopping.

PAIN MANAGEMENT

For many, managing pain is the main focus with fibromyalgia. Ginger, extra-virgin olive oil, and jalapeño peppers are some foods linked to effective pain management. Ingredients that contain omega-3 fatty acids, antioxidants, and vitamin C have been shown to reduce inflammation.

Shopping List

Fruits and Vegetables

- Asparagus, 2 bunches, about 24 spears
- Avocados, 5
- Bean sprouts, 2 cups
- Beets, 6
- Bok choy, baby, 2 pounds
- Brussels sprouts, 1 pound
- Carrots, 16
- Cauliflower, 2 heads
- Celeriac, 1 pound
- Celery stalks, 13
- Cucumber, English, 2
- Garlic cloves, 6
- Garlic, minced, ¾ cup
- Ginger, fresh, 5-inch piece
- Greens, mixed, 2 ounces
- Kale, 2 large bunches
- Leeks, 4
- Lemons, 3
- Limes, 5
- Mushrooms, button, 12 ounces
- Onion, red, 1
- Onions, sweet, 11
- Parsnips, 7
- Peppers, jalapeño, 2
- Peppers, red bell, 8
- Peppers, yellow bell, 2
- Pumpkin, 2½ pounds
- Radicchio, 1 head
- Radishes, 1 bunch (8)
- Scallions, 6
- Sweet potatoes, 5
- Swiss chard, 1 bunch
- Tomatoes, 4
- Tomatoes, cherry, 2 pints
- Zucchini, 12

Meats and Poultry

- Bacon, uncured, 8 slices
- Beef striploin steak, 1 pound
- Chicken breasts, cooked, 8 (6-ounce)
- Lamb shoulder, 2 pounds
- Pork tenderloins, 2 (12-ounce)
- Pork, ground, 3 pounds
- Turkey breast, cooked, 1 pound
- Turkey, ground, 3 pounds

Fish and Seafood

- Shrimp, peeled and deveined, 2 pounds
- Sole fillets, 4 (6-ounce)
- Whitefish fillet, 2 pounds

Fresh Herbs and Spices

- Basil, 1 small bunch
- Black pepper, freshly ground
- Cilantro, 1 bunch
- Cinnamon, ground, 1½ teaspoons
- Coriander, ground ½ teaspoon

- Cumin, ground, 2¼ teaspoons
- Himalayan salt or table salt
- Nutmeg, ground, 1½ teaspoons
- Parsley, 1 small bunch
- Red curry paste, ¼ cup
- Red pepper flakes, 1 teaspoon
- Rosemary, 1 bunch
- Thyme, 1 bunch

Dairy/Dairy Alternatives and Eggs

- Butter, grass-fed, 5 tablespoons
- Coconut milk, 9 cups
- Eggs, fresh, 25
- Eggs, hardboiled, 2
- Heavy (whipping) cream, 1¾ cups
- Kefir, coconut, ¼ cup
- Yogurt, plain, full-fat, 1 cup

Pantry Items

- Almonds, slivered, ½ cup
- Arrowroot powder, 6 tablespoons

- Broth, beef, gluten-free, sodium-free, 9½ cups
- Broth, chicken, gluten-free, sodium-free, 18¼ cups
- Cocoa powder, ¼ cup
- Coconut aminos, 5 tablespoons
- Dijon mustard, 1 teaspoon
- Oil, olive, 3¾ cups
- Oil, olive, spray
- Oil, sesame, 2 tablespoons
- Pecans, chopped, ½ cup
- Pistachios, unsalted, ½ cup
- Protein powder, plain, 2 scoops
- Sesame seeds, ¼ cup
- Sunflower seeds, ½ cup
- Tomatoes, diced, sodium-free, 2 (28-ounce) cans
- Vanilla extract, alcohol-free, 1 teaspoon
- Vinegar, apple cider, 1 tablespoon
- Xylitol, ½ cup

Other

- Edamame, frozen, 4 cups

Week 1 Meal Plan

MONDAY
Breakfast: Pumpkin, Turkey, and Swiss Chard Hash (page 72)
Lunch: Chicken Chili Soup (page 89), *double*
Dinner: Beef Chow Mein (page 188)

TUESDAY
Breakfast: Bell Pepper–Asparagus Frittata (page 76)
Lunch: Chicken Chili Soup, *leftovers*
Dinner: Pork Tenderloin with Caramelized Onions (page 179), Sweet Potato–Brussels Sprouts Toss (page 115)

WEDNESDAY

Breakfast: Chocolate-Pistachio Shake (page 64)
Lunch: Turkey–Zucchini Noodle Salad (page 90)
Dinner: Coconut-Tomato Seafood Curry (page 148), *double*

THURSDAY

Breakfast: Open-Faced Egg Sandwiches on Kale (page 124)
Lunch: Coconut-Tomato Seafood Curry, *leftovers*
Dinner: Turkey, Leek, and Pumpkin Casserole (page 174), *double*

FRIDAY

Breakfast: Turkey, Leek, and Pumpkin Casserole, *leftovers*
Lunch: Radish and Egg Salad (page 95)
Dinner: Lamb-Vegetable Stew (page 182), *double*

SATURDAY

Breakfast: Scrambled Egg and Kale (page 74)
Lunch: Lamb-Vegetable Stew, *leftovers*
Dinner: Creamy Summer Zoodles (page 134), *double*

SUNDAY

Breakfast: Sausage with Celeriac Latkes (page 75)
Lunch: Creamy Summer Zoodles, *leftovers*
Dinner: Roasted Sole with Vegetables, Garlic, and Sunflower Seeds (page 146)

snacks

Creamy Coconut Yogurt (page 214)
Cucumber Green Smoothie (page 65)
Ginger-Coconut Cookies (page 105)
½ cup almonds
1 hardboiled egg
Celery and carrot sticks
5 to 10 olives

WEEK 1

GAINING ENERGY

If you're dealing with fatigue, spinach, beef, broccoli, and citrus fruit are some foods linked to effectively managing it. Ingredients that contain protein, iron, and vitamins C and B12 have been shown to increase energy.

Shopping List

Fruits and Vegetables

- Acorn squash, 1 pound
- Asparagus, 2 pounds
- Bean sprouts, 1 cup
- Bok choy, baby, 1 pound
- Carrots, 27
- Cauliflower, 2 heads
- Celeriac, 2 whole plus 1 pound
- Celery stalks, 8
- Eggplant, 4
- Garlic cloves, 9
- Garlic, minced, 1 cup
- Ginger, fresh, 5-inch piece
- Grapefruit, ruby red, 1
- Jicama, 1
- Kale, 2 bunches
- Kohlrabi, 4
- Leeks, 4
- Lemons, 5
- Limes, 5
- Mushrooms, button, 2 ounces
- Onion, red, 1
- Onions, sweet, 13
- Parsnips, 10
- Peppers, jalapeño, 2
- Peppers, red bell, 7
- Peppers, yellow bell, 2
- Pumpkin, ½ pound (2 cups diced)
- Scallions, 9
- Spaghetti squash, 1
- Spinach, 8 ounces
- Sweet potatoes, 4
- Swiss chard, 1 bunch
- Tomatoes, 14
- Tomatoes, cherry, 4 pints
- Zucchini, 8

Meats and Poultry

- Bacon, uncured, 8 slices
- Beef, ground, 2½ pounds
- Chicken breasts, cooked, 8 (6-ounce)
- Lamb, ground, 1 pound
- Pork, ground, 1 pound
- Turkey breast, cooked, 1 pound
- Turkey, ground, 3 pounds
- Venison leg, boneless, 2 pounds

Fish and Seafood

- Shrimp (26 to 30 count), peeled and deveined, 1 pound

Fresh Herbs and Spices

- Basil, 2 large bunches
- Black pepper, freshly ground
- Cardamom, ground, ¼ teaspoon
- Cilantro, 2 bunches
- Cinnamon, ground, 1 teaspoon
- Coriander, ground, ½ teaspoon
- Cumin, ground, 1 teaspoon

WEEK 2

- Cumin seeds, 1 teaspoon
- Himalayan salt or table salt
- Mint, 1 bunch
- Nutmeg, ground, 1¾ teaspoons
- Oregano, 1 bunch
- Parsley, 1 bunch
- Red pepper flakes, 1 teaspoon
- Thyme, 1 bunch
- Turmeric, ground, 3 teaspoons

Dairy/Dairy Alternatives and Eggs

- Almond milk, unsweetened, ¾ cup
- Butter, grass-fed, 3 tablespoons
- Coconut milk, ½ cup
- Cottage cheese, full-fat, 1 cup
- Cream cheese, full-fat, 1¼ cups
- Eggs, fresh, 23
- Heavy (whipping) cream, 2½ cups
- Yogurt, plain, full-fat, 1½ cups plus 2 tablespoons

Pantry Items

- Almond butter, ½ cup
- Almond flour, 1 cup

- Almonds, sliced, ¼ cup
- Arrowroot powder, 1 teaspoon
- Broth, chicken, gluten-free, sodium-free, 38 cups (2½ gallons)
- Broth, vegetable, gluten-free, sodium-free, 12 cups (3 quarts)
- Coconut aminos, 2 tablespoons
- Dijon mustard, 2 teaspoons
- Oil, coconut, 6 tablespoons
- Oil, olive, 4 cups
- Oil, olive, spray
- Oil, sesame, 1 tablespoon
- Olives, Kalamata, sliced, ½ cup plus ¼ cup whole
- Sesame seeds, 2 tablespoons
- Sunflower seeds, 2 tablespoons
- Tomatoes, diced, sodium-free, 2 (28-ounce) cans
- Vanilla extract, alcohol-free, 1 teaspoon
- Vinegar, balsamic, ¼ cup
- Walnuts, chopped, ¾ cup
- Xylitol, 5 tablespoons

Week 2 Meal Plan

MONDAY

Breakfast: Open-Faced Egg Sandwiches on Kale (page 78)

Lunch: Basil-Tomato Salad with Herb Vinaigrette (page 93) with 1 scoop cottage cheese added

Dinner: Turkey, Leek, and Pumpkin Casserole (page 174), *double*

TUESDAY

Breakfast: Turkey, Leek, and Pumpkin Casserole, *leftovers*

Lunch: Glorious Carrot Soup (page 88), *double*

Dinner: Garlic Shrimp and Vegetables (page 140)

WEDNESDAY

Breakfast: Cinnamon Cheesecake Smoothie (page 67)
Lunch: Glorious Carrot Soup, *leftovers*
Dinner: Italian-Style Meatballs (page 191), Curried Kohlrabi (page 118)

THURSDAY

Breakfast: Bell Pepper–Asparagus Frittata (page 76)
Lunch: Turkey–Zucchini Noodle Salad (page 90)
Dinner: Winter Vegetable Stew (page 135), *double*

FRIDAY

Breakfast: Pumpkin, Turkey, and Swiss Chard Hash (page 72)
Lunch: Winter Vegetable Stew, *leftovers*
Dinner: Zucchini Pasta with Beef and Eggplant Sauce (page 187)

SATURDAY

Breakfast: Scrambled Egg and Kale (page 74)
Lunch: Asian Spinach Salad with Almond Dressing (page 92)
Dinner: Roasted Venison Leg (page 180), Mediterranean Spaghetti Squash (page 111)

SUNDAY

Breakfast: Sausage with Celeriac Latkes (page 75)
Lunch: Chicken Chili Soup (page 89), *double*
Dinner: Acorn Squash Lamb Gratin (page 184)

snacks

Grapefruit-Yogurt Smoothie (page 69)
Roasted Eggplant Dip (page 102)
Crispy Baked Parsnip Fries (page 104)
¼ cup berries
½ cup cashews
Cucumber slices
Almond butter on celery

WEEK 2

week 3

FIGHTING BRAIN FOG

Brain fog can be one of the most concerning symptoms for sufferers of fibromyalgia. Avocado, dark chocolate, and nuts are some foods linked to clearing brain fog. Ingredients that contain omega-3 fatty acids, antioxidants, and B vitamins have been shown to decrease this symptom.

Shopping List

Fruits and Vegetables

- Asparagus, 5 bunches (about 60 spears)
- Avocados, 3
- Bean sprouts, 4 cups
- Brussels sprouts, 2 pounds
- Butternut squash, 1
- Carrots, 6
- Cauliflower, 1 head
- Celeriac, 1 pound
- Cucumber, English, 1
- Garlic cloves, 8
- Garlic, minced, ¾ cup
- Ginger, fresh, 6-inch piece
- Greens, mixed, 4 to 6 ounces (4 cups)
- Kale, 1 large bunch
- Lemons, 4
- Limes, 7
- Mushrooms, button, 1 pound
- Oranges, 5
- Peppers, green bell, 2
- Peppers, jalapeño, 26
- Peppers, red bell, 18
- Peppers, yellow bell, 4
- Pumpkin, 1 pound
- Rapini, 1 bunch
- Scallions, 6
- Spinach, 2 ounces (2 cups)
- Summer squash, yellow, 2
- Sweet onions, 13
- Sweet potatoes, 6
- Swiss chard, 1 bunch
- Tangerines, 3
- Tomatoes, 4
- Tomatoes, cherry, 4 pints
- Zucchini, 2

Meats and Poultry

- Bacon, uncured, 8 slices
- Beef, ground, ¾ pound
- Chicken breasts, cooked, 4 (6-ounce)
- Chicken thighs, 1 pound
- Pork, ground, 1¾ pounds
- Turkey, ground, 5 pounds
- Venison tenderloin, 24 ounces

Fish and Seafood

- Bass fillets, 8 (6-ounce)
- Mussels, scrubbed and debearded, 1 pound
- Shrimp, peeled and deveined, 1 pound
- Whitefish, 2¼ pounds

Fresh Herbs and Spices

- Basil, 2 large bunches
- Black pepper, freshly ground
- Cardamom, ground, ½ teaspoon
- Cayenne pepper, ¼ teaspoon
- Chili powder, ½ cup

- Cilantro, 1 bunch
- Cinnamon, ground, 2⅛ teaspoons
- Cumin, ground, 1½ teaspoons
- Flaxseed, 2 tablespoons
- Himalayan salt or table salt
- Nutmeg, ground, 2 teaspoons
- Oregano, 1 small bunch
- Parsley, 1 small bunch
- Red pepper flakes, 1 teaspoon
- Rosemary, 1 bunch
- Thyme, 1 bunch
- Turmeric, ground, 1½ teaspoons

Dairy/Dairy Alternatives and Eggs

- Almond milk, unsweetened, ½ cup
- Butter, grass-fed, ¼ cup
- Coconut milk, 3 cups
- Cottage cheese, full-fat, 3 cups
- Eggs, fresh, 24
- Ghee, 2 tablespoons
- Heavy (whipping) cream, 1¼ cups
- Yogurt, plain, full-fat, 1½ cups

Pantry Items

- Almond butter, ¼ cup
- Almond flour, 1¾ cups

- Artichoke hearts, water packed, 1 (12.5-ounce) can
- Broth, chicken, gluten-free, sodium-free, ½ cup
- Broth, fish, gluten-free, sodium-free, 2 cups
- Broth, vegetable, gluten-free, sodium-free, 1 cup
- Cashews, chopped, ¾ cup
- Chickpeas, sodium-free, 1 (16-ounce) can
- Cocoa powder, ¼ cup
- Coconut aminos, 4 teaspoons
- Dijon mustard, ½ cup
- Oil, olive, 3¼ cups
- Oil, olive, spray
- Oil, sesame, ¼ cup
- Olives, Kalamata, 2 cups sliced
- Pecans, chopped, 1½ cups
- Pistachios, unsalted, 2½ cups
- Protein powder, plain, 2 scoops
- Sunflower seeds, 1 cup
- Tomatoes, diced, sodium-free, 6 (28-ounce) cans
- Vanilla extract, alcohol-free, 1 teaspoon
- Vinegar, apple cider, 2 tablespoons
- Vinegar, white, 3 cups
- Xylitol, 7 tablespoons

WEEK 3

Week 3 Meal Plan

MONDAY

Breakfast: Chocolate-Pistachio Shake (page 64)
Lunch: Chicken Chili Soup, *leftovers*
Dinner: Traditional Herbed Meatloaf (page 186), Southwestern Cauliflower Rice (page 116)

TUESDAY

Breakfast: Sausage with Celeriac Latkes (page 75)
Lunch: Avocado-Tangerine Salad (page 97), plus 1 (4-ounce) piece of fish
Dinner: Easy Chicken Pad Thai (page 168), *double*

WEDNESDAY

Breakfast: Easy Chicken Pad Thai, *leftovers*

Lunch: Refreshing Gazpacho (page 82)

Dinner: Golden Cottage Cheese–Topped Bass (page 150), *double*, Sweet Potato–Brussels Sprouts Toss (page 115), *double*

THURSDAY

Breakfast: Bell Pepper–Asparagus Frittata (page 76)

Lunch: Golden Cottage Cheese-Topped Bass, *leftovers*, Sweet Potato–Brussels Sprouts Toss, *leftovers*

Dinner: Chickpea Basil-Stuffed Peppers (page 124), *double*

FRIDAY

Breakfast: Open-Faced Egg Sandwiches on Kale (page 78)

Lunch: Chickpea Basil-Stuffed Peppers, *leftovers*

Dinner: Greek Fish Stew (page 144), *double*

SATURDAY

Breakfast: Pumpkin, Turkey, and Swiss Chard Hash (page 72)

Lunch: Greek Fish Stew, *leftovers*

Dinner: Mustard-Crusted Venison (page 181), Gingered Asparagus (page 121)

SUNDAY

Breakfast: Scrambled Egg and Kale (page 74)

Lunch: Turkey Chili (page 178), *double*

Dinner: Coconut Milk–Braised Chicken (page 173), Gingered Asparagus (page 121)

snacks

Coconut Milk–Turmeric Smoothie (page 68)

Nut-Chili Crackers (page 106)

Pretty Pickled Jalapeños (page 112)

½ orange

Broccoli and cauliflower florets

4 ounces turkey meat

½ cup full-fat cottage cheese

week 4
PROMOTING HEALTHY DIGESTION

Gut health is crucial for fighting inflammation that can contribute to many fibro-myalgia symptoms. Yogurt, cauliflower, and cumin are some foods linked to healthy digestion. Ingredients that contain fiber, probiotics, flavonoids, vitamin D, and iron have been shown to support gut health.

Shopping List

Fruits and Vegetables

- Acorn squash, 1 pound
- Asparagus, 1 bunch, about 12 spears
- Avocados, 2
- Belgian endive, 3 heads
- Bok choy, baby, 1½ pounds
- Broccoli, 1 head
- Cabbage, red, 1 head
- Carrots, 11
- Cauliflower, 6 heads
- Celeriac, 1 pound plus 1 whole
- Celery stalks, 10
- Garlic cloves, 3
- Garlic, minced, 1 cup
- Ginger, fresh, 4-inch piece
- Grapefruit, ruby red, 2
- Kale, 2 bunches
- Leeks, 4
- Lemons, 4
- Mushrooms, button, 1 cup sliced
- Onion, red, 1
- Onions, sweet, 14
- Oranges, 2
- Peppers, jalapeño, 3
- Pepper, orange bell, 1
- Peppers, red bell, 5
- Peppers, yellow bell, 2
- Pumpkin, 2½ pounds
- Radishes, 2 bunches
- Scallions, 6
- Spinach, 4 ounces
- Sweet potatoes, 2
- Swiss chard, 1 bunch
- Tomatoes, 6
- Tomatoes, cherry, 5 pints
- Zucchini, 2

Meats and Poultry

- Bacon, uncured, 8 slices
- Beef pot roast, 2 pounds
- Chicken breasts, boneless skinless, 8 (5-ounce)
- Chicken breasts, cooked, 5 (8-ounce)
- Lamb, ground, 1 pound
- Pork, ground, 1 pound
- Turkey, ground, 3 pounds

Fish and Seafood

- Flounder fillets, 8 (6-ounce)
- Shrimp, peeled and deveined, 2 pounds
- Whitefish fillets, 2 pounds

Fresh Herbs and Spices

- Basil, 1 bunch
- Black pepper, freshly ground
- Cayenne pepper, ½ teaspoon
- Cilantro, 1 bunch
- Cinnamon, ground, 1½ teaspoons

WEEK 4

- Coriander, ground, 2 teaspoons
- Cumin, ground, 4 teaspoons
- Himalayan salt or table salt
- Nutmeg, ground, 1½ teaspoons
- Oregano, 1 bunch
- Paprika, ½ teaspoon
- Parsley, 1 bunch
- Red curry paste, ¼ cup
- Red pepper flakes, 1 teaspoon
- Thyme, 1 bunch
- Turmeric, ground 1 teaspoon

Dairy/Dairy Alternatives and Eggs

- Almond milk, unsweetened, ¾ cup
- Coconut milk, 6 cups
- Cream cheese, 1½ cups
- Eggs, fresh, 21
- Ghee, ¼ cup
- Heavy (whipping) cream, ½ cup
- Yogurt, plain, full-fat, 1 cup

Pantry Items

- Almond butter, ½ cup
- Almond milk, unsweetened, ½ cup
- Almond flour, ½ cup
- Almonds, slivered, ½ cup
- Almonds, whole, ½ cup
- Broth, beef, gluten-free, sodium-free, 2 cups
- Broth, chicken, gluten-free, sodium-free, 9 cups
- Cashews, chopped, ¼ cup
- Hazelnuts, chopped, ½ cup
- Oil, coconut, 1 tablespoon
- Oil, olive, 4 cups
- Oil, olive, spray
- Pistachios, ½ cup
- Protein powder, plain, 1 scoop
- Sun-dried tomatoes, chopped, 2 cups
- Sesame seeds, ½ cup
- Sunflower seeds, 1 cup
- Tomatoes, diced, sodium-free, 5 (28-ounce) cans
- Vanilla bean, whole, 1
- Vinegar, balsamic, ½ cup
- Xylitol, 1 tablespoon

Week 4 Meal Plan

MONDAY

Breakfast: Cinnamon Cheesecake Smoothie (page 67)
Lunch: Turkey Chili, *leftovers*
Dinner: Coconut-Tomato Seafood Curry (page 148), *double*

TUESDAY

Breakfast: Bell Pepper–Asparagus Frittata (page 76)
Lunch: Coconut-Tomato Seafood Curry, *leftovers*
Dinner: Chopped Veggie Bowl (page 131), *double*

WEDNESDAY

Breakfast: Pumpkin, Turkey, and Swiss Chard Hash (page 72)
Lunch: Chopped Veggie Bowl, *leftovers*
Dinner: Chicken Cacciatore (page 172), *double*

THURSDAY

Breakfast: Open-Faced Egg Sandwiches on Kale (page 78)
Lunch: Chicken Cacciatore, *leftovers*
Dinner: Beef Pot Roast with Vegetables (page 190)

FRIDAY

Breakfast: Sausage with Celeriac Latkes (page 75)
Lunch: Fresh Summer Salad (page 91)
Dinner: Turkey, Leek, and Pumpkin Casserole (page 174), *double*

SATURDAY

Breakfast: Turkey, Leek, and Pumpkin Casserole, *leftovers*
Lunch: Avocado-Citrus Soup (page 85)
Dinner: Spice-Rubbed Flounder with Citrus Salsa (page 154), *double*, Southwestern Cauliflower Rice (page 116), *double*

SUNDAY

Breakfast: Scrambled Egg and Kale (page 74)
Lunch: Spice-Rubbed Flounder with Citrus Salsa, *leftovers*, Southwestern Cauliflower Rice, *leftovers*
Dinner: Acorn Squash Lamb Gratin (page 184)

snacks

Vanilla-Kale Smoothie (page 66)
Almond–Sesame Seed Balls (page 107)
Radish and Chicken Salad–Stuffed Endive (page 110)
1 tangerine
Radishes and carrots
½ cup plain, full-fat yogurt
Beef jerky

WEEK 4

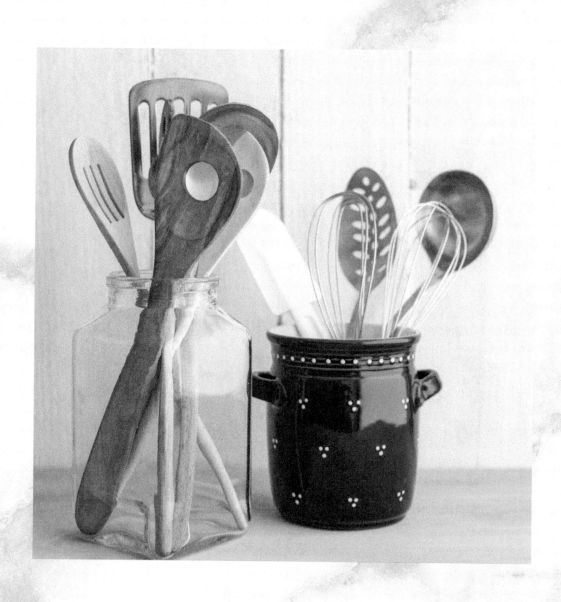

PART 3

THE RECIPES

Here, you'll find a trove of recipes. Some are contained in the meal plan, and some aren't—if you aren't pleased with a recipe on the recipe on the meal plan, feel free to swap it with one of the many others included for you. No matter which you choose, you can be sure each recipe is tailored to improve your health and wellness by fighting fibromyalgia through diet.

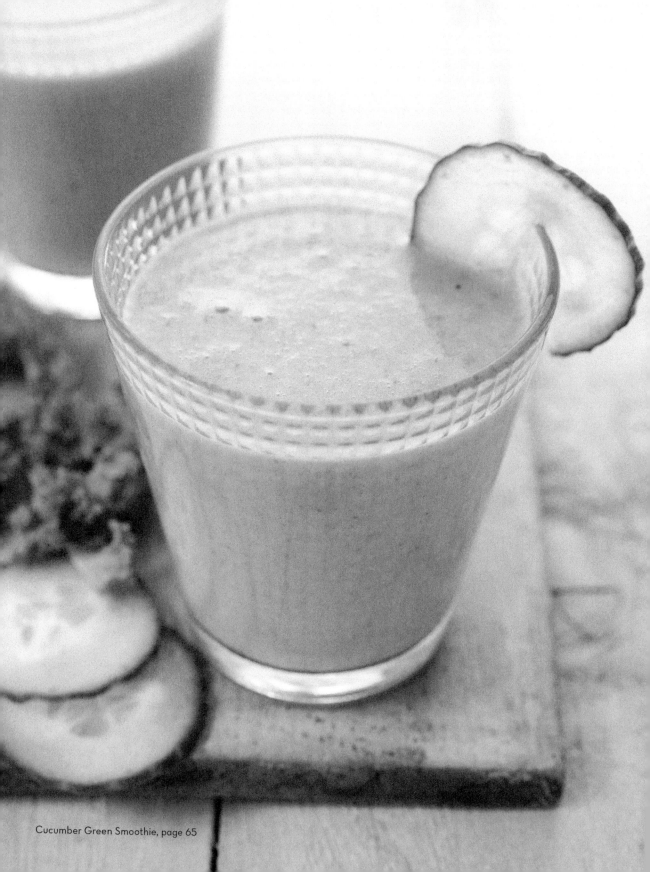

Cucumber Green Smoothie, page 65

5

smoothies & breakfasts

CHOCOLATE-PISTACHIO
SHAKE 64

CUCUMBER GREEN
SMOOTHIE 65

VANILLA-KALE
SMOOTHIE 66

CINNAMON CHEESECAKE
SMOOTHIE 67

COCONUT MILK-TURMERIC
SMOOTHIE 68

GRAPEFRUIT-YOGURT
SMOOTHIE 69

MIXED NUT PORRIDGE 70

CARAMELIZED ONION AND
SPINACH OMELET 71

PUMPKIN, TURKEY, AND
SWISS CHARD HASH 72

VEGGIE BREAKFAST
SKILLET 73

SCRAMBLED EGG
AND KALE 74

SAUSAGE WITH
CELERIAC LATKES 75

BELL PEPPER-ASPARAGUS
FRITTATA 76

SIMPLE PORK
SAUSAGES 77

OPEN-FACED
EGG SANDWICHES
ON KALE 78

CHOCOLATE-PISTACHIO SHAKE

Serves 2 | Prep time: 5 minutes | Cook time: 0 minutes

Chocolate shakes evoke visions of frosted glasses with whipped cream and a jaunty cherry on top. Although this version is not garnished with cream or fruit, it is thick and satisfyingly chocolaty. Cocoa and dark chocolate provide energy, cut through mental fog, and reduce inflammation. Cocoa is also very high in magnesium and calcium, which are crucial minerals for fibromyalgia relief and sometimes deficient in people with the condition.

1 cup coconut milk

½ cup unsalted pistachios

½ avocado, peeled and pitted

¼ cup cocoa powder

1 scoop plain protein powder

2 tablespoons xylitol

1 teaspoon alcohol-free vanilla extract

3 ice cubes

1. In a blender, combine the coconut milk, pistachios, avocado, cocoa, protein powder, xylitol, and vanilla. Blend.
2. Add the ice and blend again until thick and smooth. Serve.

Per Serving: Calories: 646; Saturated Fat: 27g; Cholesterol: 0mg; Sodium: 231mg; Calcium: 426mg; Carbohydrates: 25g; Protein: 11g

BRAIN BOOSTER

DAIRY-FREE

GLUTEN-FREE

IMMUNE BOOSTER

CUCUMBER GREEN SMOOTHIE

Serves 2 | Prep time: 5 minutes | Cook time: 0 minutes

Coconut milk makes an excellent smoothie base because it is scrumptious and rich as well as incredibly nutritious. Coconut milk contains medium chain triglycerides, which put very little strain on the liver and pancreas when converted into energy. Coconut milk is anti-inflammatory, boosts the immune system and energy levels, and fights fibro fog and fatigue with healthy fatty acids.

2 cups coconut milk

2 English cucumbers, cut into chunks

1 cup kale

1 scoop plain protein powder

1 tablespoon grated fresh ginger

½ teaspoon ground cinnamon

4 ice cubes

1. In a blender, combine the coconut milk, cucumbers, kale, protein powder, ginger, and cinnamon. Blend.
2. Add the ice and blend again until thick and smooth. Serve.

Per Serving: Calories: 549; Saturated Fat: 51g; Cholesterol: 1mg; Sodium: 83mg; Calcium: 490mg; Carbohydrates: 25g; Protein: 18g

BRAIN BOOSTER
DAIRY-FREE
GLUTEN-FREE
IMMUNE BOOSTER
PALEO-FRIENDLY

VANILLA-KALE SMOOTHIE

Serves 2 | Prep time: 5 minutes | Cook time: 0 minutes

Vanilla has such a soothing and intoxicating scent, you might find yourself sniffing this smoothie rather than drinking it! Vanilla has been considered a powerful healing agent for centuries due to its antioxidant and anti-inflammatory properties. Vanilloid—a chemical that can activate some of the same receptors as capsaicin (found in chile peppers)—helps clear mental fog and relieve stress. Vanilla can also improve digestion and reduce joint pain.

2 cups unsweetened almond milk

1 avocado, peeled and pitted

½ cup kale

1 scoop plain protein powder

Seeds from 1 vanilla bean

4 ice cubes

BRAIN BOOSTER
DAIRY-FREE
GLUTEN-FREE
IMMUNE BOOSTER
PALEO-FRIENDLY

1. In a blender, combine the almond milk, avocado, kale, protein powder, and vanilla seeds. Blend.
2. Add the ice and blend again until thick and smooth. Serve.

SIMPLIFY IT: Vanilla extract can provide an equally intense flavor if you can't find whole vanilla beans. Try 1 to 1½ teaspoons alcohol-free vanilla extract.

Per Serving: Calories: 228; Saturated Fat: 5g; Cholesterol: 32mg; Sodium: 116mg; Calcium: 310mg; Carbohydrates: 13g; Protein: 14g

CINNAMON CHEESECAKE SMOOTHIE

Serves 1 | Prep time: 10 minutes | Cook time: 0 minutes

Cinnamon is known for its ability to lower blood sugar and activate insulin receptors, and it is also an anti-inflammatory and antioxidant. For anyone living with fibromyalgia, regulating blood sugar drops and spikes is important because hypoglycemia can increase the severity of the syndrome's symptoms. Cinnamon can also reduce cellular damage and improve digestion.

¾ cup unsweetened almond milk

¼ cup cream cheese, at room temperature

2 tablespoons plain, full-fat yogurt

1 tablespoon heavy (whipping) cream

1 tablespoon xylitol

1 teaspoon ground cinnamon

2 cups ice cubes

BRAIN BOOSTER
GLUTEN-FREE
IMMUNE BOOSTER
VEGETARIAN

1. In a blender, combine the almond milk, cream cheese, yogurt, heavy cream, xylitol, and cinnamon. Blend.
2. Add the ice and blend again until thick and smooth. Serve.

COOKING TIP: You can use the ingredients right from the refrigerator, but letting the cream cheese come to room temperature gives the smoothie a nice, velvety texture. Cold cream cheese sometimes does not blend very well.

Per Serving: Calories: 314; Saturated Fat: 17g; Cholesterol: 86mg; Sodium: 314mg; Calcium: 472mg; Carbohydrates: 9g; Protein: 7g

COCONUT MILK-TURMERIC SMOOTHIE

Serves 2 | Prep time: 5 minutes | Cook time: 0 minutes

Flaxseed is the best source of plant-based omega-3 fatty acids (also known as alpha-linolenic acid, or ALA). Omega-3 fatty acids are powerful anti-inflammatories, helping reduce stiffness and joint pain. They also support healthy mental function and decrease depressive symptoms. If you don't appreciate the texture of whole flax-seed, ground flaxseed will also do the trick!

1 cup coconut milk

½ cup unsweetened almond milk

1 orange, peeled and segmented

1 cup cooked mashed carrot

1 scoop plain protein powder

2 tablespoons flaxseed

½ teaspoon ground turmeric

Pinch ground cinnamon

4 ice cubes

1. In a blender, combine the coconut milk, almond milk, orange, carrot, protein powder, flaxseed, turmeric, and cinnamon. Blend.
2. Add the ice and blend again until smooth and thick. Serve.

Per Serving: Calories: 418; Saturated Fat: 26g; Cholesterol: 1mg; Sodium: 120mg; Calcium: 580mg; Carbohydrates: 26g; Protein: 12g

BRAIN BOOSTER
DAIRY-FREE
GLUTEN-FREE
IMMUNE BOOSTER
PALEO-FRIENDLY

GRAPEFRUIT-YOGURT SMOOTHIE

Serves 2 | Prep time: 5 minutes | Cook time: 0 minutes

Grapefruit is a divine fruit—juicy and packed with nutrients. It's high in alpha hydroxy acids, which are linked to the reduction of pain, especially when combined with magnesium. Because another ingredient in this smoothie, sunflower seeds, is high in magnesium, starting the day with this filling beverage is a great strategy.

½ cup coconut milk

½ cup plain, full-fat yogurt

1 ruby red grapefruit, peeled and segmented

2 tablespoons sunflower seeds

1 tablespoon xylitol

1 teaspoon alcohol-free vanilla extract

¼ teaspoon ground nutmeg

2 cups ice cubes

1. In a blender, combine the coconut milk, yogurt, grapefruit, sunflower seeds, xylitol, vanilla, and nutmeg. Blend.
2. Add the ice and blend again until smooth. Serve.

Per Serving: Calories: 264; Saturated Fat: 14g; Cholesterol: 4mg; Sodium: 53mg; Calcium: 135mg; Carbohydrates: 16g; Protein: 7g

BRAIN BOOSTER

GLUTEN-FREE

IMMUNE BOOSTER

VEGETARIAN

MIXED NUT PORRIDGE

Serves 2 | Prep time: 15 minutes | Cook time: 10 minutes

In many cases, magnesium deficiency and fibromyalgia go hand in hand, so it is prudent to include this nutrient regularly in your diet. Magnesium can help relax muscles and nerves, improve sleep, and reduce inflammation. Consuming enough of this mineral can reduce the severity of fibromyalgia symptoms as well. The nuts and seeds in this filling porridge—almonds, cashews, and flaxseed—are very high in magnesium. Nuts and seeds are also an excellent source of B vitamins, iron, selenium, and zinc.

½ cup unsweetened almond milk

¼ cup almond flour

¼ cup chopped cashews

¼ cup flaxseed

1 tablespoon coconut flour

1 tablespoon xylitol

1 teaspoon ground cinnamon

1 cup plain, full-fat yogurt, divided

½ cup fresh blueberries, divided

BRAIN BOOSTER
GLUTEN-FREE
IMMUNE BOOSTER
VEGETARIAN

1. In a medium saucepan over medium heat, stir together the almond milk, almond flour, cashews, flaxseed, coconut flour, xylitol, and cinnamon. Cook for about 10 minutes, stirring, until warmed through. Remove from the heat and divide the porridge between 2 bowls.

2. Top with each with ½ cup yogurt and ¼ cup blueberries.

SIMPLIFY IT: Combine the nuts, seeds, xylitol, and cinnamon, and refrigerate this base mixture in a sealed jar. When you want to enjoy this European-inspired breakfast, combine some of the mixture with the milk. Stir, heat, and top with the yogurt and berries.

Per Serving: Calories: 525; Saturated Fat: 18g; Cholesterol: 8mg; Sodium: 118mg; Calcium: 280mg; Carbohydrates: 36g; Protein: 18g

CARAMELIZED ONION AND SPINACH OMELET

Serves 4 | Prep time: 15 minutes | Cook time: 23 minutes

Eggs are a wonderful source of a form of carbohydrate called D-ribose that is very effective in managing fibromyalgia pain. D-ribose can also boost energy, provide mental clarity, and improve sleep quality. Eggs are also high in omega-3 fatty acids, vitamin B_{12}, and protein—all crucial for those with fibromyalgia.

2 tablespoons extra-virgin olive oil

1 tablespoon grass-fed butter

1 sweet onion, thinly sliced

1 teaspoon minced garlic

1 cup shredded fresh spinach

12 eggs, beaten

½ teaspoon Himalayan salt or table salt

1 teaspoon freshly ground black pepper

1 cup full-fat ricotta cheese

1 tablespoon chopped fresh chives

BRAIN BOOSTER
GLUTEN-FREE
IMMUNE BOOSTER
NUT-FREE
VEGETARIAN

Per Serving: Calories: 388; Saturated Fat: 12g; Cholesterol: 528mg; Sodium: 551mg; Calcium: 210mg; Carbohydrates: 6g; Protein: 24g

1. Preheat the oven to 375°F.
2. In a large ovenproof skillet over medium-low heat, heat the olive oil and melt the butter.
3. Add the onion and garlic. Sauté for about 10 minutes, until the onion is lightly caramelized, stirring occasionally.
4. Add the spinach and sauté for 4 minutes.
5. In medium bowl, whisk the eggs, salt, and pepper. Pour the eggs into the skillet and swirl to distribute.
6. Let the eggs cook for about 5 minutes, lifting the edges to let the raw egg flow underneath the cooked egg, until almost cooked through.
7. Scatter the ricotta cheese over the top of the omelet, and place the skillet in the oven. Bake for about 4 minutes, until the top is cooked through and puffy.
8. Serve, sprinkled with the chives.

PUMPKIN, TURKEY, AND SWISS CHARD HASH

Serves 4 | Prep time: 15 minutes | Cook time: 18 minutes

Pumpkin lovers know it's a versatile vegetable that works well in both savory and sweet dishes. It is chock-full of beta-carotene and high in omega-3 and omega-6 fatty acids, calcium, magnesium, iron, potassium, and vitamins A, C, E, and K. That combination of nutrients boosts the immune system and protects against free radicals.

3 tablespoons extra-virgin olive oil

1 pound ground turkey

½ sweet onion, chopped

1 teaspoon minced garlic

2 cups shredded Swiss chard

2 cups diced cooked pumpkin

½ teaspoon ground nutmeg

Himalayan salt or table salt, for seasoning

Freshly ground black pepper, for seasoning

2 teaspoons chopped fresh thyme leaves

BRAIN BOOSTER
DAIRY-FREE
GLUTEN-FREE
IMMUNE BOOSTER
NUT-FREE
PALEO-FRIENDLY

1. In a large skillet over medium-high heat, heat the olive oil.
2. Add the turkey. Sauté for 7 to 10 minutes, breaking it up with the back of a spoon, until cooked through.
3. Add the onion and garlic, and sauté for 3 minutes more.
4. Stir in the chard, pumpkin, and nutmeg. Sauté for about 5 minutes, until the greens are wilted and the pumpkin is heated through.
5. Season the hash with salt and pepper, and serve sprinkled with thyme.

Per Serving: Calories: 366; Saturated Fat: 5g; Cholesterol: 116mg; Sodium: 225mg; Calcium: 80mg; Carbohydrates: 13g; Protein: 33g

VEGGIE BREAKFAST SKILLET

Serves 4 | Prep time: 15 minutes | Cook time: 22 minutes

This tempting breakfast choice is an inflammation-fighting masterpiece, packed with vibrant colors and interesting textures. The many colors in this dish indicate there is an extensive range of antioxidants, such as chlorophyll (green), beta-carotene (orange), lycopene (red), and lutein (yellow). The onion and garlic also add their own important antioxidants—quercetin and allicin—to the mix.

3 tablespoons extra-virgin olive oil, divided

½ sweet onion, chopped

1 teaspoon minced garlic

1 red bell pepper, chopped

1 yellow bell pepper, chopped

1 cup cauliflower florets

1 sweet potato, cubed

1 zucchini, chopped

2 cups shredded kale

Himalayan salt or table salt, for seasoning

Freshly ground black pepper, for seasoning

4 eggs

½ cup full-fat cottage cheese

1 scallion, white and green parts, chopped

BRAIN BOOSTER
GLUTEN-FREE
IMMUNE BOOSTER
NUT-FREE
VEGETARIAN

1. In a large skillet over medium-high heat, heat 4 teaspoons olive oil.
2. Add the onion and garlic. Sauté for about 3 minutes, until softened.
3. Add the red and yellow bell peppers, cauliflower, sweet potato, and zucchini. Sauté for about 12 minutes, until the vegetables are tender.
4. Add the kale and sauté for 2 minutes more. Remove the skillet from the heat, and season the veggie mixture with salt and pepper.
5. In a medium skillet over medium-high heat, heat the remaining 5 teaspoons olive oil.
6. Crack the eggs into the skillet. Cook for about 5 minutes, sunny-side up, until the whites are firm and cooked through.
7. Divide the veggie mixture among 4 plates, and top each with 1 egg and 2 tablespoons cottage cheese.
8. Garnish with the scallion and serve.

Per Serving: Calories: 291; Saturated Fat: 3g;
Cholesterol: 166mg; Sodium: 287mg; Calcium: 112mg;
Carbohydrates: 19g; Protein: 13g

SCRAMBLED EGG AND KALE

Serves 4 | Prep time: 15 minutes | Cook time: 15 minutes

Scrambled eggs get a fancy presentation with the addition of bell pepper, kale, tasty mushrooms, and a generous amount of nutmeg. Nutmeg contains an essential oil called myristicin that is an anti-inflammatory and antispasmodic, making it effective for calming the nervous system. Nutmeg stimulates blood flow to the brain providing "peace of mind" and clarity. This soothing quality can also improve sleep and concentration.

3 tablespoons extra-virgin olive oil

1 cup sliced button mushrooms

½ sweet onion, chopped

1 teaspoon minced garlic

2 cups shredded kale

1 red bell pepper, chopped

8 eggs

¼ cup heavy (whipping) cream

1 teaspoon ground nutmeg

Pinch red pepper flakes

Himalayan salt or table salt, for seasoning

Freshly ground black pepper, for seasoning

BRAIN BOOSTER
GLUTEN-FREE
IMMUNE BOOSTER
NUT-FREE
VEGETARIAN

1. In a large skillet over medium-high heat, heat the olive oil.
2. Add the mushrooms, onion, and garlic. Sauté for about 5 minutes, until the vegetables are tender.
3. Add the kale and red bell pepper and sauté for 5 minutes more.
4. In a medium bowl, whisk the eggs, heavy cream, and nutmeg. Pour the egg mixture into the skillet, and allow the mixture to cook until it sets slightly. Cook the mixture for about 5 minutes, gently stirring to scramble the eggs until cooked through.
5. Season with the red pepper flakes, salt, and pepper. Serve.

Per Serving: Calories: 281; Saturated Fat: 7g; Cholesterol: 338mg; Sodium: 202mg; Calcium: 100mg; Carbohydrates: 9g; Protein: 14g

SAUSAGE WITH CELERIAC LATKES

Serves 4 | Prep time: 15 minutes | Cook time: 10 minutes

You should be able to find celeriac, or celery root, in your supermarket's produce section. It is a fabulous source of vitamins B6, C, and K as well as calcium and fiber. Its nutrients can boost immunity, control blood sugar, and prevent nerve damage. Celeriac contains many antioxidants, and forms a strong free radical–fighting combination when mixed with onions and egg.

1 pound celeriac, peeled, shredded, and patted dry

½ cup chopped sweet onion

1 egg, lightly beaten

¼ teaspoon Himalayan salt or table salt

½ cup extra-virgin olive oil, divided

8 warm Simple Pork Sausages (page 77)

BRAIN BOOSTER
GLUTEN-FREE
IMMUNE BOOSTER
NUT-FREE
PALEO-FRIENDLY

Per Serving: Calories: 453; Saturated Fat: 6g; Cholesterol: 124mg; Sodium: 546mg; Calcium: 70mg; Carbohydrates: 13g; Protein: 33g

1. In a large bowl, stir together the celeriac, onion, egg, and salt.
2. In a large skillet over medium-high heat, heat ¼ cup olive oil.
3. Spoon ¼-cup portions of the celeriac mixture into the skillet, spreading them into 4-inch rounds. Do not crowd the skillet.
4. Fry the latkes for about 5 minutes, until golden brown and crispy on the bottom. Flip them and fry for about 5 minutes more, until the second side is golden and the middle is cooked through.
5. Transfer the latkes to a paper towel–lined plate, and repeat with the remaining ¼ cup olive oil and celeriac mixture.
6. To serve, plate 2 latkes with 2 sausages.

SIMPLIFY IT: Make the pork sausages ahead and refrigerate or freeze. Then simply thaw them or take them out of the refrigerator, and reheat them in a low-heat oven (about 300°F) for about 20 minutes.

BELL PEPPER-ASPARAGUS FRITTATA

Serves 4 | Prep time: 15 minutes | Cook time: 31 minutes

Asparagus serves up essential fibromyalgia nutrients, such as vitamins B6, C, and E, as well as calcium, beta-carotene, fiber, and magnesium. Asparagus also contains a compound called saponins and the nutrient glutathione, both powerful inflammation-fighting antioxidants.

3 tablespoons extra-virgin olive oil

½ sweet onion, chopped

2 teaspoons minced garlic

1 red bell pepper, cut into thin strips

1 yellow bell pepper, cut into thin strips

2 cups (1-inch pieces) asparagus

8 eggs

¼ cup heavy (whipping) cream

1 tablespoon chopped fresh basil leaves

Himalayan salt or table salt, for seasoning

Freshly ground black pepper, for seasoning

1 cup halved cherry tomatoes

1 scallion, white and green parts, chopped

BRAIN BOOSTER
GLUTEN-FREE
IMMUNE BOOSTER
NUT-FREE
VEGETARIAN

1. Preheat the oven to 350°F.
2. In a large ovenproof skillet over medium-high heat, heat the olive oil.
3. Add the onion and garlic. Sauté for about 3 minutes, until softened.
4. Add the red and yellow bell peppers and asparagus. Sauté for 4 minutes more.
5. While the vegetables sauté, in a medium bowl, whisk the eggs, heavy cream, and basil. Season with salt and pepper. Pour the egg mixture into the skillet, and cook for about 4 minutes, until the bottom is firm.
6. Scatter the tomatoes on top and transfer the skillet to the oven. Bake for about 20 minutes, until the eggs are cooked through.
7. Serve sprinkled with the scallion.

Per Serving: **Calories:** 301; **Saturated Fat:** 7g; **Cholesterol:** 338mg; **Sodium:** 191mg; **Calcium:** 90mg; **Carbohydrates:** 12g; **Protein:** 14g

SIMPLE PORK SAUSAGES

Serves 4 | Prep time: 10 minutes | Cook time: 15 minutes

Parsley might seem humble, but it is one of the best disease-fighting herbs. This frilly green herb has anti-inflammatory elements such as vitamin C, flavonoids, and a volatile oil called eugenol, and it improves digestion while boosting the immune system.

1 pound ground pork

¼ cup chopped sweet onion

2 teaspoons minced garlic

2 tablespoons chopped fresh parsley leaves

1 teaspoon chopped fresh basil leaves

½ teaspoon Himalayan salt or table salt

⅛ teaspoon freshly ground black pepper

Olive oil spray, for coating the patties

1. Preheat the oven to 400°F.
2. In a large bowl, mix together the pork, onion, garlic, parsley, basil, salt, and pepper until well blended.
3. Divide the pork mixture into 8 equal portions, and press them into ½-inch-thick patties.
4. Place the patties on a rimmed baking sheet, and spray them lightly with olive oil spray.
5. Bake the patties for 8 minutes. Flip and bake for 7 minutes more, until they are just cooked through. Serve.

Per Serving: Calories: 168; Saturated Fat: 2g; Cholesterol: 83mg; Sodium: 300mg; Calcium: 10mg; Carbohydrates: 1g; Protein: 30g

DAIRY-FREE

GLUTEN-FREE

IMMUNE BOOSTER

NUT-FREE

PALEO-FRIENDLY

OPEN-FACED EGG
SANDWICHES ON KALE

Serves 4 | Prep time: 15 minutes | Cook time: 18 minutes

Dark leafy greens are absolutely bursting with nutrients, phytonutrients, and anti-oxidants. Kale is incredibly high in vitamins A, B, C, E, and K as well as folate, fiber, magnesium, potassium, calcium, iron, and zinc. Folate is crucial for energy production because it is needed for red blood cells, which oxygenate the body, to form and grow. Tomatoes also boost energy because they are a terrific source of biotin, a B vitamin that helps enzymes work effectively in the body.

8 uncured bacon slices

4 cups chopped deribbed kale

2 teaspoons minced garlic

4 eggs

1 cup halved cherry tomatoes

Himalayan salt or table salt, for seasoning

Freshly ground black pepper, for seasoning

1 scallion, white and green parts, chopped

BRAIN BOOSTER
DAIRY-FREE
GLUTEN-FREE
IMMUNE BOOSTER
NUT-FREE
PALEO-FRIENDLY

1. In a large skillet over medium-high heat, cook the bacon for about 6 minutes, until crispy.

2. Transfer the bacon to a paper towel-lined plate. Reserve 3 tablespoons bacon drippings from the skillet, leaving 1 tablespoon in the skillet. Return the skillet to the heat.

3. Add the kale and garlic to the skillet. Cook for about 7 minutes, tossing, until the greens are wilted. Remove the skillet from the heat and set aside.

4. In a medium skillet over medium-high heat, heat the reserved 2 tablespoons bacon drippings.

5. Crack the eggs into the skillet. Fry for about 5 minutes, sunny-side up, until the whites are firm and cooked through.
6. Arrange the kale on 4 plates and top each with ¼ cup cherry tomatoes and 2 bacon slices.
7. Arrange 1 egg on each stack and season with salt and pepper.
8. Garnish with chopped scallion and serve.

A CLOSER LOOK: Uncured bacon is just like regular bacon except it is not cured with nitrates or nitrites. Instead it is cured with celery extract or plain salt, which means the meat's taste is apparent rather than artificial flavors.

Per Serving: Calories: 267; Saturated Fat: 6g; Cholesterol: 184mg; Sodium: 287mg; Calcium: 120mg; Carbohydrates: 10g; Protein: 12g

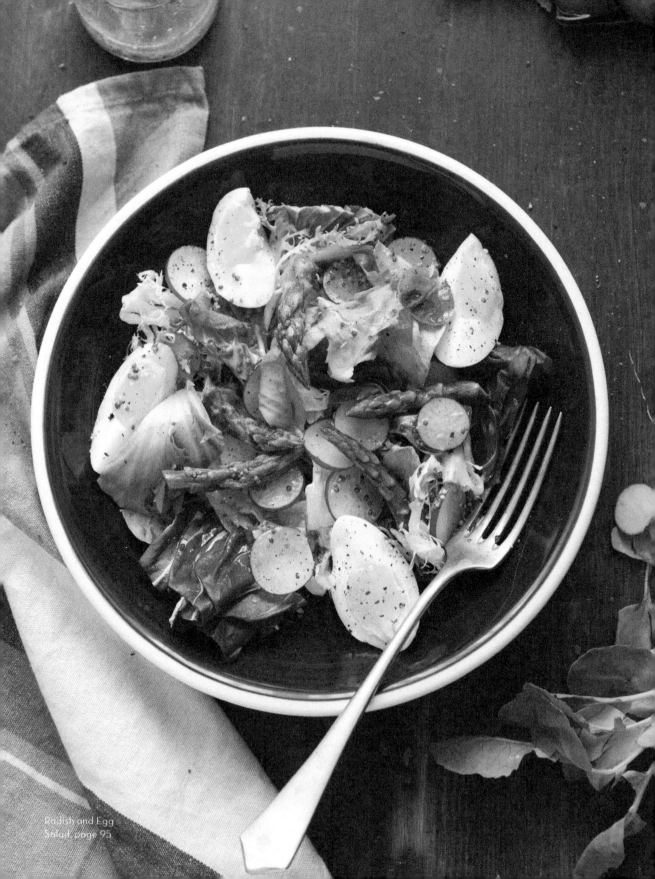

Radish and Egg
Salad, page 95

6

soups & salads

REFRESHING GAZPACHO 82

COLD CUCUMBER-DILL
SOUP 83

THAI COCONUT
MILK SOUP 84

AVOCADO-CITRUS SOUP 85

TOMATO-JALAPEÑO
SOUP 86

ROASTED CAULIFLOWER-
BROCCOLI SOUP 87

GLORIOUS CARROT
SOUP 88

CHICKEN CHILI SOUP 89

TURKEY-ZUCCHINI
NOODLE SALAD 90

FRESH SUMMER SALAD 91

ASIAN SPINACH SALAD
WITH ALMOND
DRESSING 92

BASIL-TOMATO SALAD
WITH HERB
VINAIGRETTE 93

CURRIED CABBAGE
SALAD 94

RADISH AND
EGG SALAD 95

PESTO-KALE SALAD 96

AVOCADO-TANGERINE
SALAD 97

KALE-MIXED
VEGETABLE SALAD 98

REFRESHING GAZPACHO

Serves 4 | Prep time: 20 minutes, plus chilling time | Cook time: 0 minutes

Gazpacho is a cold soup packed with healthy vegetables and flavored with fresh, fragrant herbs such as basil. Basil has traditionally been used in herbal medicine for digestive issues such as cramps and nausea, but it is also a powerful anti-inflammatory. Basil contains a chemical compound called eugenol that acts similarly to pain medications such as Tylenol. This herb inhibits the same enzyme those medications do, so pain is diminished.

3 tomatoes, quartered

2 garlic cloves

1 English cucumber, cut into chunks

1 yellow bell pepper, quartered

1 jalapeño pepper, quartered

½ sweet onion

¼ cup fresh cilantro leaves

1 cup gluten-free sodium-free vegetable broth

1 avocado, peeled, pitted, and quartered

Zest of 1 lime

Juice of 1 lime

2 tablespoons extra-virgin olive oil

½ teaspoon Himalayan salt or table salt

Freshly ground black pepper, for seasoning

1 cup plain, full-fat yogurt

¼ cup fresh basil leaves

1. In a food processor, combine the tomatoes, garlic, cucumber, yellow bell pepper, jalapeño, onion, and cilantro. Pulse until the vegetables are coarsely chopped.
2. Add the vegetable broth, avocado, lime zest and juice, olive oil, and salt. Pulse until smooth.
3. Season with pepper and stir to combine.
4. Transfer the soup to a container, and refrigerate for at least 1 hour to mellow the flavors.
5. Serve the soup topped with ¼ cup yogurt and a sprinkling of basil for each serving.

Per Serving: Calories: 254; Saturated Fat: 4g; Cholesterol: 4mg; Sodium: 301mg; Calcium: 150mg; Carbohydrates: 18g; Protein: 7g

BRAIN BOOSTER
GLUTEN-FREE
IMMUNE BOOSTER
NUT-FREE
VEGETARIAN

COLD CUCUMBER-DILL SOUP

Serves 2 | Prep time: 15 minutes | Cook time: 0 minutes

Cucumber is about 95 percent water, but it is also packed with fibromyalgia-fighting nutrients such as fiber, vitamin C, silica, potassium, magnesium, and many anti-oxidants such as quercetin, beta-carotene, luteolin, and kaempferol. Silica supports connective tissue; vitamin C is a powerful antioxidant that can reduce inflammation; fiber promotes a healthy digestive system and helps lower blood sugar.

2 English cucumbers, cut into chunks

1 celery stalk, cut into chunks

1 avocado, peeled and pitted

Zest of 1 lemon

Juice of 1 lemon

½ cup chopped fennel

1 garlic clove

2 tablespoons coconut oil

2 cups gluten-free, sodium-free chicken broth

Himalayan salt or table salt, for seasoning

Freshly ground black pepper, for seasoning

1 tablespoon chopped fresh dill

BRAIN BOOSTER
DAIRY-FREE
GLUTEN-FREE
IMMUNE BOOSTER
PALEO-FRIENDLY

1. In a food processor, combine the cucumber, celery, avocado, lemon zest and juice, fennel, garlic, and coconut oil. Pulse until very finely chopped.
2. Add the chicken broth and purée until smooth.
3. Transfer the soup to a serving bowl, and season with salt and pepper.
4. Serve the soup topped with dill.

COOKING TIP: Lime juice and zest can be used instead of lemon depending on your preference; just use 2 limes instead of 1 lemon. Citrus is crucial to brighten the flavor and provide the acid required to prevent the avocado from oxidizing to an ugly grayish color.

Per Serving: Calories: 339; Saturated Fat: 10g; Cholesterol: 0mg; Sodium: 221mg; Calcium: 100mg; Carbohydrates: 23g; Protein: 7g

THAI COCONUT MILK SOUP

Serves 4 | Prep time: 20 minutes | Cook time: 33 minutes

This festive and rich soup gets its beautiful color courtesy of sweet potatoes, which also add heaps of antioxidants and nutrients. Sweet potatoes contain 400 percent of the recommended daily amount (RDA) of vitamin A and 50 percent of the RDA of manganese and vitamin C. Sweet potatoes can help stabilize blood sugar and reduce inflammation. The bright color of this root vegetable indicates a huge amount of beta-carotene, and the addition of coconut milk, a healthy fat, ensures increased uptake of beta-carotene in the body.

2 tablespoons coconut oil

½ sweet onion, chopped

2 teaspoons minced garlic

3 cups gluten-free, sodium-free chicken broth

2 cups coconut milk

4 sweet potatoes, cut into chunks

1 teaspoon red pepper flakes

Himalayan salt or table salt, for seasoning

Freshly ground black pepper, for seasoning

¼ cup shredded unsweetened coconut

2 tablespoons chopped fresh cilantro leaves

BRAIN BOOSTER
DAIRY-FREE
GLUTEN-FREE
IMMUNE BOOSTER
PALEO-FRIENDLY

1. In a large saucepan over medium-high heat, heat the coconut oil.
2. Add the onion and garlic. Sauté for about 3 minutes, until softened.
3. Stir in the chicken broth, coconut milk, sweet potatoes, and red pepper flakes. Bring to a boil, reduce the heat to low, and simmer for about 30 minutes until the sweet potatoes are tender.
4. Transfer to a food processor, and purée until very smooth. Return the soup to the saucepan, and season with salt and pepper.
5. Serve topped with the coconut and cilantro.

Per Serving: Calories: 546; Saturated Fat: 31g; Cholesterol: 6mg; Sodium: 125mg; Calcium: 50mg; Carbohydrates: 51g; Protein: 7g

AVOCADO-CITRUS SOUP

Serves 4 | Prep time: 15 minutes | Cook time: 15 minutes

Jalapeño pepper adds a lovely heat to this soup but does not overpower the other ingredients. These lively little peppers fight inflammation and contain the phyto-chemical capsaicin, which inhibits the neuropeptide substance P that transmits pain signals to the central nervous system from the sensory nerves and is also linked to stress and anxiety regulation. The hotter the pepper, the more capsaicin it contains, so if heat is something you enjoy in your food, try fiery habaneros or serranos.

3 tablespoons extra-virgin olive oil

1 sweet onion, chopped

1 jalapeño pepper, chopped

2 teaspoons minced garlic

6 cups gluten-free, sodium-free chicken broth

2 cups diced cooked chicken

2 cups diced canned sodium-free tomatoes

Zest of 1 lemon

Juice of 1 lemon

1 avocado, peeled, pitted, and diced

1 tablespoon chopped fresh cilantro leaves

Himalayan salt or table salt, for seasoning

Freshly ground black pepper, for seasoning

¼ cup plain, full-fat yogurt

BRAIN BOOSTER
GLUTEN-FREE
IMMUNE BOOSTER
NUT-FREE

1. In a large saucepan over medium-high heat, heat the olive oil.
2. Add the onion, jalapeño, and garlic. Sauté for about 3 minutes, until softened.
3. Stir in the chicken broth, chicken, tomatoes, and lemon zest and juice. Bring to a boil, reduce the heat to low, and simmer for about 10 minutes, until heated through.
4. Stir in the avocado and cilantro.
5. Season the soup with salt and pepper, and serve topped with yogurt.

SIMPLIFY IT: Cooked chicken can keep in the refrigerator in sealed containers for up to 4 days. Poach several breasts at the beginning of the week, and chop them to have ready for recipes such as this.

Per Serving: Calories: 362; Saturated Fat: 5g; Cholesterol: 55mg; Sodium: 227mg; Calcium: 60mg; Carbohydrates: 14g; Protein: 26g

TOMATO-JALAPEÑO SOUP

Serves 4 | Prep time: 15 minutes | Cook time: 23 minutes

This delicious vibrant and fiery soup is seasoned with apple cider vinegar, which has both culinary and health benefits. Along with brightening flavors, apple cider vinegar can help alleviate many symptoms associated with fibromyalgia. The malic acid in it can help reduce muscle pain because the acid binds to toxins found in the muscles, allowing the body to eliminate them. Apple cider vinegar also contains potassium, which fights lactic acid buildup, which can cause fatigue.

3 tablespoons extra-virgin olive oil

1 sweet onion, chopped

1 jalapeño pepper, chopped

2 teaspoons minced garlic

2 (28-ounce) cans sodium-free diced tomatoes

2 cups gluten-free sodium-free chicken broth

1 red bell pepper, chopped

1 cup sun-dried tomatoes

2 tablespoons apple cider vinegar

3 tablespoons chopped fresh basil leaves

Himalayan salt or table salt, for seasoning

Freshly ground black pepper, for seasoning

1. In a large saucepan over medium-high heat, heat the olive oil.
2. Add the onion, jalapeño, and garlic. Sauté for about 3 minutes until softened.
3. Stir in the tomatoes, chicken broth, red bell pepper, sun-dried tomatoes, cider vinegar, and basil. Bring the soup to a boil, reduce the heat to low, and simmer for 20 minutes.
4. Transfer the soup to a food processor, and pulse until smooth.
5. Return the soup to the saucepan, and season it with salt and pepper. Serve.

Per Serving: Calories: 269; Saturated Fat: 3g; Cholesterol: 6mg; Sodium: 421mg; Calcium: 150mg; Carbohydrates: 31g; Protein: 8g

BRAIN BOOSTER

DAIRY-FREE

GLUTEN-FREE

IMMUNE BOOSTER

NUT-FREE

PALEO-FRIENDLY

ROASTED CAULIFLOWER-BROCCOLI SOUP

Serves 4 | Prep time: 20 minutes | Cook time: 45 minutes

Cruciferous vegetables are one category of foods to eat every day. Not only are they an incredible source of phytonutrients, vitamins C and K, and fiber, cruciferous vegetables, such as broccoli and cauliflower, also contain a compound called ascorbigen. Ascorbigen can help reduce tenderness and pain, which is one reason these vegetables are so important in a fibromyalgia diet.

1 head cauliflower, cut into florets
1 head broccoli, cut into florets
1 sweet onion, cut into eight wedges
3 garlic cloves, lightly crushed
3 tablespoons extra-virgin olive oil
Himalayan salt or table salt, for seasoning
Freshly ground black pepper, for seasoning
6 cups gluten-free sodium-free chicken broth
½ cup heavy (whipping) cream
1 teaspoon ground nutmeg

BRAIN BOOSTER
GLUTEN-FREE
IMMUNE BOOSTER
NUT-FREE

1. Preheat the oven to 400°F.
2. Line a rimmed baking sheet with parchment paper.
3. Arrange the cauliflower, broccoli, onion, and garlic on the prepared sheet, and drizzle with the olive oil. Season the vegetables with salt and pepper.
4. Roast them for about 30 minutes, until tender and lightly caramelized, stirring once. Transfer to a food processor.
5. Add the chicken broth and purée. (Do this in batches if necessary, adding both vegetables and broth to each batch.) Transfer the puréed soup to a large saucepan over medium heat.
6. Whisk in the heavy cream and nutmeg. Cook until heated through and serve.

Per Serving: Calories: 269; Saturated Fat: 7g; Cholesterol: 58mg; Sodium: 311mg; Calcium: 80mg; Carbohydrates: 14g; Protein: 13g

GLORIOUS CARROT SOUP

Serves 4 | Prep time: 10 minutes | Cook time: 33 minutes

This soup showcases carrots, a stellar source of vitamins A and K, beta-carotene, and fiber. Turmeric, a heady counterpoint to carrots, is often touted as a fibromyalgia super spice because it contains curcumin, the source of the spice's distinctive yellow color. Curcumin is an extremely powerful anti-inflammatory and antioxidant offering many benefits for the body, including improving insulin resistance and reduced inflammation, especially when consumed with black pepper. Black pepper increases curcumin's bioavailability, making it quickly and efficiently absorbed by the body.

3 tablespoons extra-virgin olive oil

1 sweet onion, chopped

2 teaspoons minced garlic

8 carrots, cut into chunks

8 cups gluten-free, sodium-free chicken broth

1 teaspoon ground turmeric

½ teaspoon ground cumin

Himalayan salt or table salt, for seasoning

Freshly ground black pepper, for seasoning

½ cup heavy (whipping) cream

1 tablespoon chopped fresh parsley leaves

BRAIN BOOSTER
GLUTEN-FREE
IMMUNE BOOSTER
NUT-FREE

1. In a large saucepan over medium-high heat, heat the olive oil.
2. Add the onion and garlic. Sauté for about 3 minutes, until softened.
3. Stir in the carrots, chicken broth, turmeric, and cumin. Bring the soup to a boil, reduce the heat to low, and simmer for about 30 minutes, until the carrots are tender.
4. Transfer the soup to a blender, and blend until very smooth.
5. Return the soup to the saucepan, and season with salt and pepper.
6. Whisk in the heavy cream, and serve topped with parsley.

A CLOSER LOOK: Carrots can cut the risk of glaucoma, protect against cardiovascular disease, and support the immune system.

Per Serving: Calories: 288; Saturated Fat: 7g; Cholesterol: 21mg; Sodium: 225mg; Calcium: 80mg; Carbohydrates: 22g; Protein: 4g

CHICKEN CHILI SOUP

Serves 4 | Prep time: 25 minutes | Cook time: 25 minutes

This delicious soup has a healthy dose of garlic, that fragrant ingredient popular in many cuisines worldwide. Garlic also holds a special place in herbal medicine circles as an aid for treating different conditions, due to its antioxidant, antiviral, and antibacterial properties. Garlic is a rich source of allicin, a sulfur-containing compound that can reduce inflammation, and many other nutrients that can lower blood pressure, detoxify the body, and even fight the common cold.

3 tablespoons extra-virgin olive oil

3 celery stalks, chopped

1 sweet onion, chopped

1 jalapeño pepper, minced

1 tablespoon minced garlic

1 tablespoon grated fresh ginger

8 cups gluten-free, sodium-free chicken broth

4 cups diced cooked chicken

2 cups shredded baby bok choy

2 carrots, thinly sliced

1 red bell pepper, thinly sliced

¼ cup chopped fresh cilantro leaves

Pinch red pepper flakes

2 scallions, white and green parts, sliced on a bias

½ cup plain, full-fat yogurt

1. In a large stockpot over medium-high heat, heat the olive oil.
2. Add the celery, onion, jalapeño, garlic, and ginger. Sauté for about 6 minutes, until softened.
3. Stir in the chicken broth, chicken, bok choy, carrots, red bell pepper, cilantro, and red pepper flakes. Bring the soup to a boil, reduce the heat to low, and simmer for about 15 minutes, until the vegetables are tender.
4. Serve topped with scallions and yogurt.

Per Serving: Calories: 443; Saturated Fat: 5g; Cholesterol: 160mg; Sodium: 428mg; Calcium: 140mg; Carbohydrates: 14g; Protein: 54g

BRAIN BOOSTER
GLUTEN-FREE
IMMUNE BOOSTER
NUT-FREE

TURKEY-ZUCCHINI
NOODLE SALAD

Serves 4 | Prep time: 25 minutes | Cook time: 0 minutes

This salad features many ingredients that contain nutrients important for managing fibromyalgia. Ginger and garlic contain antioxidants; carrots are high in vitamin A; red bell peppers are a source of vitamin C; sesame seeds are rich in omega-3 fatty acids; turkey provides protein, which repairs damaged muscles, producing pain relief.

For the dressing

¼ cup gluten-free, sodium-free chicken broth

¼ cup freshly squeezed lime juice

1 tablespoon xylitol

1 tablespoon minced fresh ginger

1 tablespoon coconut aminos

2 teaspoons minced garlic

Pinch red pepper flakes

For the salad

1 pound cooked turkey breast, shredded

4 cups zucchini noodles

1 carrot, shredded

1 red bell pepper, thinly sliced

1 cup bean sprouts

¼ cup chopped fresh cilantro leaves

2 tablespoons sesame seeds

BRAIN BOOSTER
DAIRY-FREE
GLUTEN-FREE
IMMUNE BOOSTER

To make the dressing

In small bowl, whisk the chicken broth, lime juice, xylitol, ginger, coconut aminos, garlic, and red pepper flakes until well combined. Set aside.

To make the salad

1. In large bowl, toss the turkey, zucchini noodles, carrot, red bell pepper, bean sprouts, and cilantro until well distributed.
2. Pour the dressing over the salad and toss until well combined.
3. Chill and serve topped with sesame seeds.

A CLOSER LOOK: Sesame seeds come in different colors that taste the same but provide different looks. In your local grocery store, you can find black, golden, and red seeds. Choose whichever color you like for the salad.

Per Serving: Calories: 198; Saturated Fat: 1g; Cholesterol: 49mg; Sodium: 654mg; Calcium: 80mg; Carbohydrates: 17g; Protein: 24g

FRESH SUMMER SALAD

Serves 4 | Prep time: 30 minutes | Cook time: 0 minutes

This lively salad is dressed with ubiquitous olive oil, treasured in most kitchens for its health benefits, ability to combine well with other ingredients, and moderately high smoke point. Olive oil is high in a hormone called DHEA, which can counteract damage caused by inflammation. Olive oil is also rich in vitamin E, an antioxidant that supports brain health, improves endurance, and balances hormones.

2 zucchini, diced

2 carrots, diced

1 red bell pepper, thinly sliced

1 yellow bell pepper, thinly sliced

1 orange bell pepper, thinly sliced

1 cup halved cherry tomatoes

1 cup cauliflower florets

1 cup shredded fresh spinach

½ red onion, thinly sliced

½ cup chopped fresh parsley leaves

¼ cup balsamic vinegar

¼ cup extra-virgin olive oil

2 (8-ounce) cooked boneless skinless
   chicken breasts, thinly sliced

Freshly ground black pepper, for seasoning

1. In a large bowl, toss together the zucchini; carrots; red, yellow, and orange bell peppers; tomatoes; cauliflower; spinach; red onion; parsley; balsamic vinegar; and olive oil until very well mixed.

2. Arrange the salads on 4 plates and top each with chicken. Season with pepper and serve.

Per Serving: Calories: 408; Saturated Fat: 5g; Cholesterol: 101mg; Sodium: 152mg; Calcium: 80mg; Carbohydrates: 18g; Protein: 37g

BRAIN BOOSTER

DAIRY-FREE

GLUTEN-FREE

IMMUNE BOOSTER

NUT-FREE

PALEO-FRIENDLY

ASIAN SPINACH SALAD WITH ALMOND DRESSING

Serves 4 | Prep time: 25 minutes | Cook time: 0 minutes

You may already know how rich in iron spinach is, but you might not know that iron is a valuable nutrient for fibromites. Iron deficiency, or anemia, can cause fatigue, headaches, and a slew of other symptoms. Many people with fibromyalgia suffer from anemia and don't know it. Eating iron-rich dark leafy greens can be proactive in addressing this.

For the dressing

½ cup almond butter

Zest of 2 limes

Juice of 2 limes

1 tablespoon coconut aminos

1 tablespoon grated fresh ginger

1 tablespoon sesame oil

2 teaspoons xylitol

For the salad

4 cups fresh spinach

2 carrots, shredded

1 cup chopped kale

1 red bell pepper, thinly sliced

1 cup shredded jicama

1 scallion, white and green parts, chopped

2 tablespoons chopped fresh cilantro leaves

¼ cup sliced toasted almonds

To make the dressing

In a small bowl, whisk the almond butter, lime zest and juice, coconut aminos, ginger, sesame oil, and xylitol until blended. Set aside.

To make the salad

1. In a large bowl, toss together the spinach, carrots, kale, red bell pepper, jicama, scallion, and cilantro.
2. Add the dressing and toss to coat. Serve topped with the almonds.

Per Serving: Calories: 136; Saturated Fat: 2g; Cholesterol: 0mg; Sodium: 60mg; Calcium: 90mg; Carbohydrates: 15g; Protein: 5g

BRAIN BOOSTER

DAIRY-FREE

GLUTEN-FREE

IMMUNE BOOSTER

VEGETARIAN

BASIL-TOMATO SALAD
WITH HERB VINAIGRETTE

Serves 4 | Prep time: 15 minutes | Cook time: 0 minutes

This Mediterranean-style salad is very nutritionally supportive of fibromyalgia sufferers. Polyphenols in olives can reduce inflammation in the body by lowering the blood levels of C-reactive protein. Tomatoes, onion, basil, and parsley are packed with antioxidants and vitamins that can reduce the severity of fibromyalgia symptoms.

For the dressing

½ cup extra-virgin olive oil

¼ cup freshly squeezed lemon juice

2 teaspoons Dijon mustard

1 teaspoon minced garlic

¼ cup chopped fresh parsley leaves

For the salad

8 tomatoes, sliced

¼ cup thinly sliced red onion

½ cup sliced Kalamata olives

½ cup shredded fresh basil leaves

Himalayan salt or table salt, for seasoning

Freshly ground black pepper, for seasoning

BRAIN BOOSTER

GLUTEN-FREE

IMMUNE BOOSTER

NUT-FREE

PALEO-FRIENDLY

VEGETARIAN

To make the dressing

In a small bowl, whisk the olive oil, lemon juice, mustard, garlic, and parsley until well blended. Set aside.

To make the salad

1. Arrange the tomatoes on a serving plate.
2. Scatter the red onion, olives, and basil evenly over the tomatoes.
3. Season the salad with salt and pepper and drizzle with the dressing. Serve.

COOKING TIP: For a truly spectacular salad, use multicolored heirloom tomatoes, such as red, yellow, orange, pink, and purple. Arrange the different colors to create gorgeous patterns on the plate.

Per Serving: Calories: 291; Saturated Fat: 5g; Cholesterol: 0mg; Sodium: 251mg; Calcium: 60mg; Carbohydrates: 12g; Protein: 3g

CURRIED CABBAGE SALAD

Serves 6 | Prep time: 20 minutes, plus 1 hour chilling time | Cook time: 0 minutes

This is really just a fancy coleslaw recipe, but that doesn't mean it isn't utterly delicious. The salad base is two types of the fibromyalgia-friendly cruciferous vegetable, cabbage, although you could use just one type in a pinch. The cashews add crunch and a healthy amount of protein and zinc. Many people who experience stress and anxiety have low levels of zinc, so replenishing this mineral is beneficial.

For the dressing
¾ cup plain, full-fat yogurt

2 tablespoons freshly squeezed lemon juice

1 tablespoon curry powder

1 tablespoon xylitol

¼ teaspoon ground turmeric

Himalayan salt or table salt, for seasoning

For the salad
½ head napa cabbage, shredded

½ head red cabbage, shredded

2 carrots, shredded

2 parsnips, shredded

½ red onion, very thinly sliced

½ cup chopped cashews

To make the dressing

In a small bowl, whisk the yogurt, lemon juice, curry powder, xylitol, and turmeric. Season with salt and set aside.

To make the salad

1. In a large bowl, toss together the napa and red cabbage, carrots, parsnips, red onion, and cashews.
2. Add the dressing and stir to coat. Refrigerate the salad for at least 1 hour to let the flavors mellow. Serve.

Per Serving: Calories: 245; Saturated Fat: 3g; Cholesterol: 3mg; Sodium: 208mg; Calcium: 280mg; Carbohydrates: 34g; Protein: 10g

BRAIN BOOSTER
GLUTEN-FREE
IMMUNE BOOSTER
VEGETARIAN

RADISH AND EGG SALAD

Serves 4 | Prep time: 25 minutes | Cook time: 0 minutes

This pretty salad will make you smile when you see the colors and textures on the plate. Radicchio adds a gorgeous deep red to the dish and has a lovely bite to it. It is a rich source of fiber, antioxidants, phytonutrients, B-vitamins, and vitamins A, C, E, and K. One of the most effective components of radicchio for a fibromyalgia diet is an antimalarial agent known as lactucopicrin *(intybin), a sesquiterpene lactone. It produces a sedative and analgesic (painkiller) effect.*

For the dressing

3 tablespoons extra-virgin olive oil

1 tablespoon apple cider vinegar

1 teaspoon Dijon mustard

½ teaspoon minced garlic

Himalayan salt or table salt, for seasoning

Freshly ground black pepper, for seasoning

For the salad

2 cups mixed greens

2 cups radicchio, torn into pieces

1 cup sliced radishes

1 cup (1-inch pieces) asparagus

2 hardboiled eggs, quartered

BRAIN BOOSTER
GLUTEN-FREE
IMMUNE BOOSTER
NUT-FREE
VEGETARIAN

To make the dressing

In a small bowl, whisk the olive oil, cider vinegar, mustard, and garlic. Season with salt and pepper and set aside.

To make the salad

1. In a medium bowl, toss the greens and radicchio with half the dressing until well coated. Arrange on 4 plates.
2. Top each salad with ¼ cup radishes, ¼ cup asparagus, and 2 egg quarters.
3. Drizzle the salads with the remaining dressing and serve.

SIMPLIFY IT: Hardboiled eggs are a perfect snack choice and wonderful shredded or sliced in salads and other dishes. Boil a dozen or so, and keep them refrigerated, unpeeled, for up to 1 week.

Per Serving: Calories: 435; Saturated Fat: 8g; Cholesterol: 137mg; Sodium: 267mg; Calcium: 94mg; Carbohydrates: 11g; Protein: 30g

PESTO-KALE SALAD

Serves 4 | Prep time: 20 minutes | Cook time: 0 minutes

This surprisingly elegant-looking dish, mostly in pale greens and bits of gold from the pine nuts, is one of those salads that is incredibly quick to put together but looks like you spent hours getting it just perfect. Pine nuts are not actually nuts; they are the seeds of pine trees, which is apparent in their flavor. Pine nuts are very high in magnesium, monounsaturated fat, protein, and iron—nutrients that boost energy levels and fight fatigue. These pretty seeds are also the source of many inflammation-fighting antioxidants.

5 cups chopped kale

2 cups cauliflower florets

1 cup chopped water-packed canned
    artichoke hearts

½ cup Herb and Roasted Red Pepper
    Pesto (page 208)

6 beets, peeled and shredded

1 scallion, white and green parts, thinly sliced

¼ cup pine nuts

1. In a large bowl, toss together the kale, cauliflower, artichoke hearts, and pesto until well coated.
2. Arrange the salad on 4 plates, and top each equally with beets, scallion, and pine nuts. Serve.

Per Serving: Calories: 332; Saturated Fat: 3g; Cholesterol: 3mg; Sodium: 396mg; Calcium: 270mg; Carbohydrates: 32g; Protein: 12g

BRAIN BOOSTER

DAIRY-FREE

GLUTEN-FREE

IMMUNE BOOSTER

NUT-FREE

PALEO-FRIENDLY

VEGETARIAN

AVOCADO-TANGERINE SALAD

Serves 4 | Prep time: 20 minutes | Cook time: 0 minutes

Segments of vibrant tangerine, pale green chunks of avocado, mounds of fresh dark leafy greens, and a tangy ginger-citrus dressing make a spectacular-looking and tasting starter or light lunch. Avocado contains a slew of nutrients that can ease fibromyalgia symptoms, such as healthy fats, fiber, vitamins E and K, and several B vitamins along with protein, magnesium, and iron. Avocados can fight fatigue and inflammation, reduce blood pressure and stress, and improve gut health.

For the dressing

¼ cup freshly squeezed orange juice

2 tablespoons apple cider vinegar

1 teaspoon grated orange zest

1 teaspoon freshly grated ginger

¼ cup extra-virgin olive oil

For the salad

4 cups mixed greens

2 cups rapini

3 tangerines, peeled and segmented

1 avocado, peeled, pitted, and diced

1 cup sunflower seeds

BRAIN BOOSTER
DAIRY-FREE
GLUTEN-FREE
IMMUNE BOOSTER
NUT-FREE
PALEO-FRIENDLY
VEGETARIAN

To make the dressing

1. In a small bowl whisk the orange juice, cider vinegar, orange zest, and ginger.
2. Whisk in the olive oil until it emulsifies. Set aside.

To make the salad

1. In a large bowl, toss the greens and rapini with half the dressing until well coated.
2. Arrange the greens on a serving plate, and top with the tangerines, avocado, and sunflower seeds.
3. Drizzle with the remaining dressing and serve.

Per Serving: Calories: 372; Saturated Fat: 4g; Cholesterol: 0mg; Sodium: 35mg; Calcium: 70mg; Carbohydrates: 27g; Protein: 7g

KALE-MIXED VEGETABLE SALAD

Serves 4 | Prep time: 20 minutes | Cook time: 0 minutes

The combination of vegetables in this dish can be changed depending on your personal preference or what is in season where you live. The lightly herbed dressing will complement many different choices. Two types of cruciferous vegetables, cauliflower and broccoli, and a heap of kale ensure this salad is very high in the nutrients and antioxidants that can make a difference in your health. The topping of rich sunflower seeds adds vitamins B₁ and E, selenium, and magnesium. These seeds can help fight inflammation and calm the pain in nerves and muscles.

BRAIN BOOSTER
DAIRY-FREE
GLUTEN-FREE
IMMUNE BOOSTER
NUT-FREE
PALEO-FRIENDLY
VEGETARIAN

For the dressing

½ cup extra-virgin olive oil

¼ cup balsamic vinegar

1 teaspoon chopped fresh basil leaves

½ teaspoon chopped fresh oregano leaves

Himalayan salt or table salt, for seasoning

Freshly ground black pepper, for seasoning

For the salad

4 cups chopped kale

1 cup halved cherry tomatoes

1 cup (1-inch) broccoli florets

½ cup quartered radishes

½ English cucumber, diced

½ cup chopped cauliflower

¼ cup sunflower seeds

To make the dressing

1. In a small bowl, whisk the olive oil, balsamic vinegar, basil, and oregano.
2. Season with salt and pepper and set aside.

To make the salad

1. In a large bowl, toss together the kale, cherry tomatoes, broccoli, radishes, cucumber, and cauliflower.
2. Add the dressing and toss to combine.
3. Top the salad with the sunflower seeds. Serve.

SIMPLIFY IT: Double or triple the dressing recipe and refrigerate it in a sealed jar or container for all your salad needs. Shake it before dressing this tempting salad combination.

Per Serving: Calories: 297; Saturated Fat: 4g; Cholesterol: 0mg; Sodium: 108mg; Calcium: 120mg; Carbohydrates: 14g; Protein: 4g

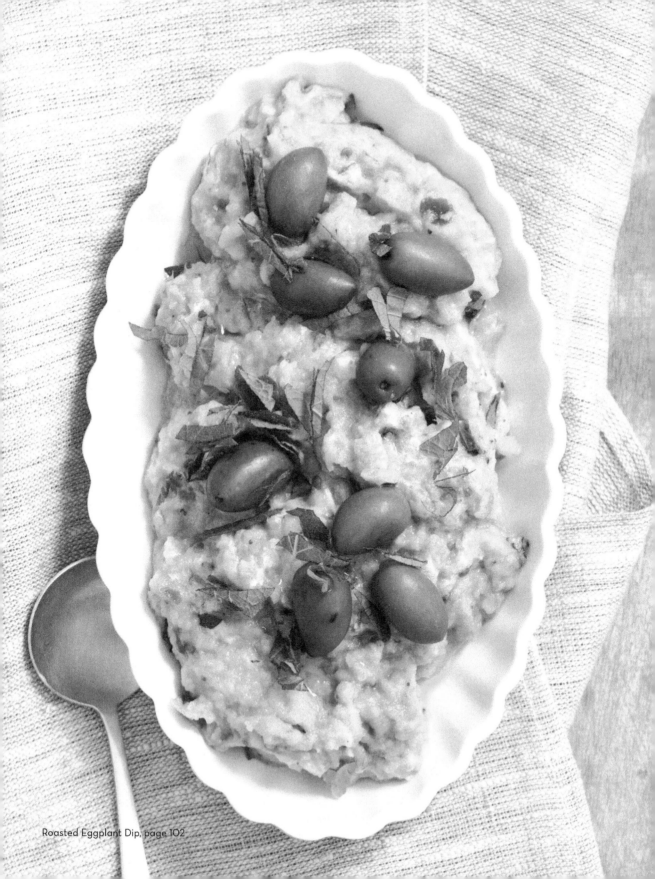

Roasted Eggplant Dip, page 102

7
snacks & sides

ROASTED EGGPLANT
DIP 102

LETTUCE SPRING
ROLLS 103

CRISPY BAKED
PARSNIP FRIES 104

GINGER-COCONUT
COOKIES 105

NUT-CHILI CRACKERS 106

ALMOND-SESAME
SEED BALLS 107

BLUEBERRY-ALMOND
SCONES 108

RADISH AND CHICKEN
SALAD-STUFFED
ENDIVE 110

MEDITERRANEAN
SPAGHETTI SQUASH 111

PRETTY PICKLED
JALAPEÑOS 112

THYME-BAKED
ARTICHOKES 114

SWEET POTATO-BRUSSELS
SPROUTS TOSS 115

SOUTHWESTERN
CAULIFLOWER RICE 116

BALSAMIC-BRAISED
ONIONS 117

CURRIED KOHLRABI 118

HOMEMADE
SAUERKRAUT 120

GINGERED ASPARAGUS 121

ROASTED EGGPLANT DIP

Makes 4 cups | Prep time: 15 minutes | Cook time: 1 hour

This delicious dip is, basically, a version of the traditional baba ganoush recipe with a few additions, such as oregano, onion, and olives. The eggplants in this recipe are not peeled—and for good reason. The skin contains a phytonutrient called nasunin. *This phytonutrient is good for brain health because it protects the lipids found in the cell membranes of brain cells, which in turn can protect the cells from free radicals.*

3 eggplants, sliced

1 sweet onion, cut into eight wedges

4 garlic cloves, crushed

¼ cup extra-virgin olive oil

Juice of 1 lemon

Himalayan salt or table salt, for seasoning

¼ cup Kalamata olives

1 tablespoon chopped fresh oregano leaves

BRAIN BOOSTER
DAIRY-FREE
GLUTEN-FREE
IMMUNE BOOSTER
NUT-FREE
PALEO-FRIENDLY
VEGETARIAN

1. Preheat the oven to 350°F.
2. Line a rimmed baking sheet with parchment paper.
3. Arrange the eggplant slices in a single layer on the prepared sheet. Scatter the onion and garlic on the eggplant, and drizzle with olive oil and lemon juice.
4. Roast the vegetables for about 1 hour, until the eggplant is very tender.
5. Let the vegetables cool on the baking sheet.
6. Transfer the cooled vegetables to a food processor along with any juices on the sheet, and purée until chopped but not entirely smooth.
7. Transfer the mixture to a container and season with salt.
8. Top with olives and oregano and serve. Refrigerate the dip for up to 3 days.

Per Serving (½ cup): Calories: 120; Saturated Fat: 1g; Cholesterol: 0mg; Sodium: 73mg; Calcium: 40mg; Carbohydrates: 15g; Protein: 3g

LETTUCE SPRING ROLLS

Serves 4 | Prep time: 30 minutes | Cook time: 0 minutes

Lettuce rolls are a staple snack food in many Asian cultures because they are delicious, lettuce is inexpensive, and you can carry them around easily. Lettuce is surprisingly high in many nutrients such as vitamins A and K, folate, fiber, and potassium. Lettuce can reduce inflammation and boost energy, especially when stuffed with antioxidant-packed red and yellow bell peppers and carrots.

1 red bell pepper, thinly sliced

1 yellow bell pepper, thinly sliced

2 cups shredded cabbage

1 English cucumber, julienned

2 carrots, julienned

½ cup fresh cilantro leaves, minced

8 large Boston lettuce leaves

1¼ cup Sesame-Lemon Dressing (page 211)

BRAIN BOOSTER

DAIRY-FREE

GLUTEN-FREE

IMMUNE BOOSTER

NUT-FREE

PALEO-FRIENDLY

VEGETARIAN

1. In a large bowl, toss together the red and yellow bell peppers, cabbage, cucumber, carrots, and cilantro until well combined.

2. Place the lettuce leaves on a clean work surface. Divide the vegetable mixture evenly among them. Fold the sides of the leaves over the filling, and roll up from the bottom to form tight cylinders.

3. Serve the rolls with the dressing.

COOKING TIP: The combination of vegetables in these crunchy wraps can be changed depending on what is in your refrigerator or what your favorites are. Shredded broccoli stalks, radishes, bok choy, parsnips, and scallions can all be wrapped and dipped.

Per Serving: Calories: 285; Saturated Fat: 14g; Cholesterol: 0mg; Sodium: 118mg; Calcium: 120mg; Carbohydrates: 20g; Protein: 7g

CRISPY BAKED PARSNIP FRIES

Serves 4 | Prep time: 10 minutes | Cook time: 30 minutes

Parsnips look like pale cream-colored carrots, which is not surprising considering they are closely related to the more brightly colored vegetable. Parsnips are high in fiber and vitamins C, E, and K as well as calcium, iron, and a multitude of anti-oxidants. This vegetable is anti-inflammatory, supports healthy digestion, and boosts the metabolism for weight loss goals. Parsnips are relatively high in natural sugar, so they caramelize beautifully when baked in a high-heat oven.

6 parsnips, peeled and cut into ½-inch batons about 3 inches long

2 tablespoons arrowroot powder

¼ cup extra-virgin olive oil

½ teaspoon Himalayan salt or table salt

DAIRY-FREE
GLUTEN-FREE
IMMUNE BOOSTER
NUT-FREE
PALEO-FRIENDLY
VEGETARIAN

1. Preheat the oven to 400°F.
2. Line a large rimmed baking sheet with parchment paper.
3. Place the parsnips in a plastic freezer bag, and add the arrowroot powder. Seal the bag and shake to coat the vegetables. Transfer the coated parsnips to a fine-mesh strainer, and shake to remove any excess arrowroot.
4. In a large bowl, toss the coated parsnips with the olive oil and salt. Spread the fries on the prepared sheet in a single layer
5. Bake for about 30 minutes, turning once, until crispy and golden. Serve.

Per Serving: Calories: 266; Saturated Fat: 2g; Cholesterol: 0mg; Sodium: 254mg; Calcium: 70mg; Carbohydrates: 38g; Protein: 4g

GINGER-COCONUT COOKIES

Makes 16 | Prep time: 15 minutes | Cook time: 12 minutes

Ginger cookies are a comforting snack that would not be out of place in a bear-shaped cookie jar in your grandmother's kitchen. The eggs and butter add a fair amount of protein to the finished treat, and the ginger and coconut flour are very high in anti-inflammatory properties. Coconut flour can be tricky to use if you have never baked with it before, so stick precisely to the recipe or your cookies may not turn out well.

4 eggs

¼ cup (½ stick) grass-fed butter, softened

2 tablespoons xylitol

2 teaspoons freshly grated ginger

½ cup coconut flour

Pinch Himalayan salt or table salt

GLUTEN-FREE
IMMUNE BOOSTER
VEGETARIAN

1. Preheat the oven to 350°F.
2. Line a rimmed baking sheet with parchment paper.
3. In a large bowl, beat the eggs with an electric hand mixer for about 5 minutes, until they are thick and pale yellow.
4. Beat in the butter, xylitol, and ginger until smooth.
5. Stir in the coconut flour and salt until well mixed.
6. Drop the batter by tablespoons onto the prepared sheet about 1 inch apart.
7. Bake for 10 to 12 minutes, until golden.
8. Cool the cookies on a wire rack, and store in a sealed container at room temperature for up to 4 days.

Per Serving (2 cookies): Calories: 93; Saturated Fat: 5g; Cholesterol: 97mg; Sodium: 107mg; Calcium: 10mg; Carbohydrates: 2g; Protein: 4g

NUT-CHILI CRACKERS

Makes 24 | Prep time: 25 minutes | Cook time: 10 minutes

Pecans are packed with many antioxidants including ellagic acid, oleic acid, vitamin E, beta-carotene, and lutein—all powerful inflammation fighters. Almonds are rich in folate and healthy omega-3 fatty acids. The combination of the two nuts creates a perfect energy-boosting snack. Cayenne is a stellar source of capsaicin and beta-carotene, a carotenoid that is converted to vitamin A in the body. These components are natural pain relievers and fight inflammation.

¾ cup almond flour

½ cup ground pecans

1 teaspoon xylitol

⅛ teaspoon cayenne pepper

2 tablespoons extra-virgin olive oil

2 egg whites

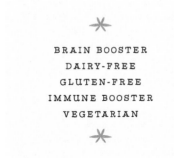

BRAIN BOOSTER
DAIRY-FREE
GLUTEN-FREE
IMMUNE BOOSTER
VEGETARIAN

SIMPLIFY IT: Nut flours can be made at home with a food processor or blender, but you can buy both products in the local supermarket. Avoid products sold in bulk, because they can be rancid.

1. Preheat the oven to 350°F.
2. Line a 9-by-13-inch baking dish with parchment paper.
3. In a medium bowl, stir together the almond flour, pecans, xylitol, and cayenne until well mixed.
4. Make a well in the center and pour in the olive oil and egg whites. Stir to form a stiff dough, and press the dough evenly in the baking dish.
5. Using a paring knife, cut the dough into 24 squares.
6. Bake for about 10 minutes, until the crackers are golden brown.
7. Cool the crackers in the baking dish. Refrigerate the cooled crackers in a sealed container for up to 1 week.

Per Serving (2 crackers): **Calories: 134; Saturated Fat: 3g; Cholesterol: 0mg; Sodium: 6mg; Calcium: 16mg; Carbohydrates: 2g; Protein: 2g**

ALMOND-SESAME SEED BALLS

Makes 16 balls | Prep time: 15 minutes, plus 1 hour chilling time | Cook time: 0 minutes

If you need a blast of energy or a mental boost during your day, savor a couple of these tender nutty treats and enjoy the benefits. Most of the ingredients in these balls are healthy fats, with the cinnamon helping stabilize your blood sugar. The nuts and seeds are potent anti-inflammatories and can help clear the fibro fog that can be an issue for many people with fibromyalgia.

½ cup almond butter

½ cup pistachios

½ cup almonds

½ cup sesame seeds

1 tablespoon coconut oil

½ teaspoon ground cinnamon

BRAIN BOOSTER

DAIRY-FREE

GLUTEN-FREE

IMMUNE BOOSTER

PALEO-FRIENDLY

VEGETARIAN

1. In a blender, combine the almond butter, pistachios, almonds, sesame seeds, coconut oil, and cinnamon. Pulse until the nuts are finely chopped and the mixture sticks together.

2. Scoop the mixture by spoonfuls, and roll each spoonful into a ball. Place the balls in a container, and refrigerate for about 1 hour until the balls firm up. Keep refrigerated in a sealed container for up to 1 week.

Per Serving (2 balls): Calories: 127; Saturated Fat: 3g; Cholesterol: 0mg; Sodium: 21mg; Calcium: 110mg; Carbohydrates: 5g; Protein: 4g

BLUEBERRY-ALMOND SCONES

Makes 8 | Prep time: 10 minutes | Cook time: 25 minutes

Almond flour creates a tender-crumbed scone with a distinctive nutty flavor. Almonds are also antioxidant rich and anti-inflammatory; they have no glycemic impact on blood sugar and so can help stabilize it. They are also high in magnesium, protein, and omega-3 fatty acids, which are important nutrients for fibromyalgia management. The combination of these nutrients can lessen muscle pain and improve mental clarity. Seven almonds contain a full serving of calcium, so enjoying these scones can help balance magnesium and calcium in the body.

1¾ cups almond flour

¾ cup arrowroot powder, divided,
   plus extra for dusting the work surface

2 tablespoons xylitol

1 tablespoon gluten-free baking powder

¼ teaspoon fine Himalayan salt or table salt

1 egg

¼ cup grass-fed butter, melted

1 cup fresh blueberries

BRAIN BOOSTER
GLUTEN-FREE
IMMUNE BOOSTER
VEGETARIAN

1. Preheat the oven to 350°F.
2. Line a rimmed baking sheet with parchment paper.
3. In a medium bowl, stir together the almond flour, ½ cup arrowroot powder, xylitol, baking powder, and salt.
4. In a small bowl, whisk the egg and melted butter.
5. Add the wet ingredients to the dry ingredients, and stir just until mixed.
6. In another small bowl, toss together the blueberries and remaining ¼ cup arrowroot powder. Add the coated berries to the batter.

7. Dust your work surface with a little arrowroot powder, and press the dough into a flat disk about 1 inch thick. Cut the dough into 8 equal wedges, and place them on the prepared sheet about 2 inches apart.

8. Bake the scones for about 20 to 25 minutes until tender and golden brown.

9. Remove from the oven and cool on a wire rack. Serve.

Per Serving (2 scones): Calories: 199; Saturated Fat: 8g; Cholesterol: 71mg; Sodium: 256mg; Calcium: 190mg; Carbohydrates: 12g; Protein: 4g

COOKING TIP: Always use fresh blueberries for these scones or you might end up with purple scones instead of a light gold color. Frozen blueberries cannot be stirred into dough without breaking down.

RADISH AND CHICKEN SALAD-STUFFED ENDIVE

Serves 4 | Prep time: 20 minutes | Cook time: 0 minutes

Serve these gorgeous creations as an appetizer at your next party. A member of the daisy family, Belgian endive is an elegant tapered lettuce. Endive is a fabulous source of vitamins B6 and C, potassium, calcium, magnesium, and copper. Its bitter taste comes from a compound called intybin, which is a digestive aid and can help clear toxins from the liver and blood. Healthy liver function is crucial for fighting inflammation and boosting the immune system.

1 cup shredded baby bok choy

1 cup shredded radishes

2 scallions, white and green parts, thinly sliced

1 cup diced cooked chicken breast

½ cup plain, full-fat yogurt

¼ cup chopped cashews

1 tablespoon chopped fresh parsley leaves

1 tablespoon freshly squeezed lemon juice

16 large Belgian endive leaves

1. In a large bowl, toss together the bok choy, radishes, scallions, chicken, yogurt, cashews, parsley, and lemon juice.

2. Spoon the filling into the endive leaves and serve.

Per Serving (4 stuffed leaves): Calories: 123; Saturated Fat: 2g; Cholesterol: 21mg; Sodium: 67mg; Calcium: 130mg; Carbohydrates: 7g; Protein: 10g

BRAIN BOOSTER
GLUTEN-FREE
IMMUNE BOOSTER

MEDITERRANEAN SPAGHETTI SQUASH

Serves 4 | Prep time: 15 minutes | Cook time: 35 minutes

Squash is better known nutritionally for its beta-carotene, but this lovely vegetable is also an excellent source of vitamin B_{12}. B vitamins can boost energy and help the body respond better to stress. Fibromites can experience stress, exhaustion, and anxiety, so consuming enough B vitamins, such as B_{12}, can reduce these symptoms.

3 tablespoons extra-virgin olive oil, divided

1 spaghetti squash, halved lengthwise, seeds and pulp removed

2 tomatoes, diced

1 scallion, white and green parts, chopped

Juice of ½ lemon

1 tablespoon chopped fresh oregano leaves

1 tablespoon chopped fresh basil leaves

Himalayan salt or table salt, for seasoning

Freshly ground black pepper, for seasoning

1. Preheat the oven to 400°F.
2. Lightly oil a rimmed baking sheet with 1 tablespoon olive oil.
3. Place the squash, cut-side down, on the prepared sheet, and bake for about 35 minutes, until tender.
4. Let the squash cool for 10 minutes, and scrape out the strands with a fork into a medium bowl.
5. Stir in the remaining 2 tablespoons olive oil, tomatoes, scallion, lemon juice, oregano, and basil.
6. Season with salt and pepper. Serve.

Per Serving: Calories: 130; Saturated Fat: 3g; Cholesterol: 0mg; Sodium: 88mg; Calcium: 60mg; Carbohydrates: 14g; Protein: 3g

BRAIN BOOSTER
DAIRY-FREE
GLUTEN-FREE
IMMUNE BOOSTER
NUT-FREE
PALEO-FRIENDLY
VEGETARIAN

PRETTY PICKLED JALAPEÑOS

Makes 3 (1-pint) jars | Prep time: 15 minutes, plus 20 minutes pickling time
Cook time: 5 minutes

Pickling food items to preserve vegetables and fruits for the colder winter months is an easy culinary technique that has been around for centuries. The white vinegar in this recipe is high in bioactive components that make it a potent antioxidant and antimicrobial. Vinegar can help lower blood sugar, reduce inflammation, and increase nutrient absorption.

3 cups white vinegar

3 cups water

6 garlic cloves, quartered

2 tablespoons xylitol

2 tablespoons Himalayan salt or table salt

24 jalapeño peppers, thinly sliced

3 fresh thyme sprigs

BRAIN BOOSTER
DAIRY-FREE
GLUTEN-FREE
IMMUNE BOOSTER
NUT-FREE
VEGETARIAN

1. Preheat the oven to 225°F.
2. In a large saucepan over high heat, stir together the vinegar, water, garlic, xylitol, and salt. Bring to a boil.
3. Stir in the jalapeños, and remove the saucepan from the heat. Let the mixture sit for 20 minutes.
4. While the jalapeños sit, arrange 3 clean 1-pint jars and their lids on a rimmed baking sheet, and place them in the oven. Heat the jars for 20 minutes. Remove them carefully to a heatproof board.
5. Using tongs, transfer the jalapeño slices and garlic to the jars, packing them in tightly but leaving about 1-inch of headspace at the top.

6. Add a thyme sprig to each jar, and pour in enough brining liquid to fill the jars. Seal the jars tightly with the lids. Wait for the lids to seal completely—you will hear a popping sound. Refrigerate your pickled jalapeños for up to 2 months.

A CLOSER LOOK: Thyme is a fabulous source of vitamins A, B₆, C, E, and K as well as iron, manganese, calcium, and potassium. Thyme is also very high in healthy volatile oils and flavonoids.

Per Serving (¼ pint): Calories: 22; Saturated Fat: 0g; Cholesterol: 0mg; Sodium: 1,098mg; Calcium: 10mg; Carbohydrates: 4g; Protein: 1g

THYME-BAKED ARTICHOKES

Serves 4 | Prep time: 10 minutes | Cook time: 25 minutes

Artichokes look like strange otherworldly flowers with their spiky concentric leaves and stems. If you have never cooked a whole artichoke, this construction might look a little intimidating, but don't let that deter you. The combination of the artichokes, antioxidant-rich garlic and thyme, and a generous splash of inflammation-fighting lemon juice is very beneficial and delicious.

4 artichokes, washed thoroughly,
   stems and 1 inch of the tops removed
¼ cup chopped fresh thyme leaves
3 tablespoons ghee
2 garlic cloves
Juice of 1 lemon
Himalayan salt or table salt, for seasoning
Freshly ground black pepper, for seasoning

BRAIN BOOSTER
GLUTEN-FREE
IMMUNE BOOSTER
NUT-FREE
PALEO-FRIENDLY
VEGETARIAN

Per Serving: Calories: 173; Saturated Fat: 5g; Cholesterol: 16mg; Sodium: 213mg; Calcium: 130mg; Carbohydrates: 20g; Protein: 7g

1. Preheat the oven to 400°F.
2. Bring a large pot of water to a boil, and reduce the heat to a simmer.
3. Blanch the artichokes in the simmering water for about 15 minutes until tender and the leaves can be removed easily. Remove the vegetables from the water and place them, stem-side up, on a clean kitchen towel.
4. In a blender, combine the thyme, ghee, garlic, and lemon juice. Pulse until smooth.
5. Cut the artichokes into quarters, and place them on a rimmed baking sheet.
6. Brush the artichokes with the thyme mixture, and bake them for about 10 minutes, until lightly browned.
7. Season with salt and pepper and serve.

A CLOSER LOOK: Artichokes are a variety of thistle, not really a vegetable. They are high in vitamins A, D, E, and K as well as iron, calcium, potassium, and zinc. Artichokes can help protect against cardiovascular disease, diabetes, cancer, and digestive issues.

SWEET POTATO-BRUSSELS SPROUTS TOSS

Serves 6 | Prep time: 20 minutes | Cook time: 40 minutes

Brussels sprouts are a member of the cruciferous vegetable family, so it is one of the vegetables recommended to enjoy daily to manage fibromyalgia. Brussels sprouts are incredibly high in vitamin K, specifically vitamin K_1 (both forms of the vitamin are essential to health). Vitamin K can help improve all symptoms of fibromyalgia, so including foods high in this vitamin in your meals every day can produce significant improvement in your condition.

3 sweet potatoes, diced

1 pound Brussels sprouts, ends trimmed

3 tablespoons extra-virgin olive oil

1 teaspoon ground cinnamon

¼ teaspoon ground cumin

⅛ teaspoon Himalayan salt or table salt

½ cup chopped pecans

BRAIN BOOSTER
DAIRY-FREE
GLUTEN-FREE
IMMUNE BOOSTER
PALEO-FRIENDLY
VEGETARIAN

1. Preheat the oven to 400°F.
2. In a large bowl, toss together the sweet potatoes, Brussels sprouts, olive oil, cinnamon, cumin, and salt. Arrange the vegetables on a rimmed baking sheet.
3. Roast for about 40 minutes, tossing several times, until the vegetables are tender and lightly caramelized.
4. Remove the vegetables from the oven, and transfer to a serving bowl. Add the pecans and toss to mix. Serve.

Per Serving: Calories: 293; Saturated Fat: 2g; Cholesterol: 0mg; Sodium: 67mg; Calcium: 60mg; Carbohydrates: 36g; Protein: 6g

SOUTHWESTERN CAULIFLOWER RICE

Serves 4 | Prep time: 15 minutes | Cook time: 10 minutes

When riced, or finely chopped, cauliflower has a texture similar to rice and is just as versatile a side dish. Cauliflower is rich in a vitamin-like substance called coenzyme Q10 (CoQ10), also known as ubiquinone. CoQ10 is an effective antioxidant and low levels in the body can cause cell damage. People with fibromyalgia have been shown to have lower concentrations of CoQ10 in their blood, so replenishing it through food sources is important.

2 tablespoons ghee

1 sweet onion, chopped

1 jalapeño pepper, chopped

2 teaspoons minced garlic

½ teaspoon ground turmeric

½ cup gluten-free, sodium-free chicken broth

1 head cauliflower, finely chopped (see Tip)

1 tomato, diced

Himalayan salt or table salt, for seasoning

Freshly ground black pepper, for seasoning

2 tablespoons chopped fresh cilantro leaves

BRAIN BOOSTER
DAIRY-FREE
GLUTEN-FREE
IMMUNE BOOSTER
NUT-FREE
PALEO-FRIENDLY

1. In a large skillet over medium-high heat, melt the ghee.
2. Add the onion, jalapeño, garlic, and turmeric. Sauté for about 4 minutes, until softened.
3. Stir in the chicken broth, and bring to a simmer.
4. Add the cauliflower and tomato, stir to combine, cover the skillet, and simmer for about 5 minutes, until the cauliflower is tender.
5. Season the mixture with salt and pepper. Top with cilantro and serve.

COOKING TIP: If you make a great deal of cauliflower rice, investing in a food processor might save some time and effort. Cut the cauliflower into large florets and pulse them until they are the texture of short-grain rice.

Per Serving: Calories: 103; Saturated Fat: 4g; Cholesterol: 16mg; Sodium: 90mg; Calcium: 30mg; Carbohydrates: 8g; Protein: 2g

BALSAMIC-BRAISED ONIONS

Serves 4 | Prep time: 5 minutes | Cook time: 35 minutes

Despite their strong flavor, onions have a great deal of natural sugar, so they caramelize beautifully. Balsamic vinegar speeds this process along and adds a luscious richness to the dish. Historically, balsamic vinegar was often used to treat various ailments because it is very high in antioxidants. It can reduce inflammation, act as a pain reliever, promote effective digestion, and enhance insulin sensitivity.

4 sweet onions, quartered

3 tablespoons olive oil

¼ cup balsamic vinegar

1 tablespoon chopped fresh basil leaves

⅛ teaspoon Himalayan salt or table salt

⅛ teaspoon freshly ground black pepper

DAIRY-FREE
GLUTEN-FREE
IMMUNE BOOSTER
NUT-FREE
PALEO-FRIENDLY
VEGETARIAN

1. Preheat the oven to 400°F.
2. Arrange the onions in a 9-by-9-inch baking dish, and drizzle them with the olive oil and balsamic vinegar.
3. Cover the baking dish, and place it in the oven to braise for about 20 minutes, stirring occasionally, until the onions are tender.
4. Remove the cover, and continue to braise for about 15 minutes more, until the liquid evaporates and a thick sweet glaze forms.
5. Sprinkle the onions with the basil, salt, and pepper and serve.

Per Serving: Calories: 137; Saturated Fat: 2g; Cholesterol: 0mg; Sodium: 64mg; Calcium: 30mg; Carbohydrates: 10g; Protein: 2g

CURRIED KOHLRABI

Serves 4 | Prep time: 15 minutes | Cook time: 30 minutes

Kohlrabi, that curious-looking knobby purple or green bulb, is worth a second look when perusing the produce aisles at the grocery store. Kohlrabi has more than 100 percent of the RDA of vitamin C and is rich in potassium, fiber, and iron along with many other vitamins and minerals. This tasty vegetable can boost the immune system and metabolism, support healthy nerve and muscle function, and improve digestion. When you add inflammation-fighting turmeric to the dish, you have a powerful combination to fight fibromyalgia symptoms.

2 whole kohlrabi, peeled and diced

1 tablespoon minced garlic, divided

3 tablespoons extra-virgin olive oil, divided

1 sweet onion, diced

2 cups gluten-free, sodium free chicken broth

1 teaspoon ground turmeric

½ teaspoon ground coriander

Pinch ground cardamom

Pinch Himalayan salt or table salt

¼ cup chopped walnuts

2 tablespoons shredded basil leaves

BRAIN BOOSTER
DAIRY-FREE
GLUTEN-FREE
IMMUNE BOOSTER
PALEO-FRIENDLY
VEGETARIAN

1. Preheat the oven to 400°F.
2. In a large bowl, toss the kohlrabi and 1 teaspoon garlic with 2 tablespoons olive oil. Spread the vegetables on a rimmed baking sheet.
3. Bake for about 20 minutes, until the vegetables are just cooked through.
4. While the kohlrabi bakes, in a large saucepan over medium-high heat, heat the remaining tablespoon olive oil.
5. Add the remaining 2 teaspoons garlic and the onion. Sauté for about 3 minutes until tender.

6. Stir in the chicken broth, turmeric, coriander, cardamom, and salt. Bring to a boil, reduce the heat to low, and simmer for about 10 minutes to mellow the liquid.
7. Stir in the roasted kohlrabi, and simmer for about 10 minutes more, until it is very tender, stirring occasionally.
8. Serve topped with walnuts and basil.

Per Serving: Calories: 218; Saturated Fat: 2g; Cholesterol: 0mg; Sodium: 153mg; Calcium: 73mg; Carbohydrates: 16g; Protein: 6g

HOMEMADE SAUERKRAUT

Makes 2 to 3 pints | Prep time: 10 minutes, plus several days' fermenting time
Cook time: 0 minutes

Sauerkraut can be a bit of an acquired taste. This recipe is naturally fermented and can help restore gut health, which improves digestion and reduces inflammation. Fermented products like sauerkraut can be beneficial for relieving pain and general aches, and clearing fibro fog. Mix the sauerkraut with mashed sweet potatoes or other root vegetables to create a filling casserole.

1 head green cabbage, finely shredded, reserving 6 to 8 large, whole leaves
2 tablespoons Himalayan salt or table salt

BRAIN BOOSTER
DAIRY-FREE
GLUTEN-FREE
IMMUNE BOOSTER
NUT-FREE
PALEO-FRIENDLY
VEGETARIAN

Per Serving (1 cup): Calories: 22; Saturated Fat: 0g; Cholesterol: 0mg; Sodium: 786mg; Calcium: 40mg; Carbohydrates: 5g; Protein: 2g

1. Layer the shredded cabbage in a large bowl, and sprinkle with the salt.
2. Press and toss the mixture with your hands until the liquid in the cabbage starts to purge.
3. Place the reserved leaves over the cabbage mixture, and cover the bowl with plastic wrap, with the wrap touching the surface of the leaves.
4. Arrange some weights, such as large cans of vegetables, on the plastic wrap, and leave the bowl out at room temperature for 24 hours.
5. The liquid should rise above the shredded cabbage. If not, stir in a little more salt. Let the sauerkraut sit for 2 to 6 days, until it is well fermented and smells tangy.
6. Pack it into sterilized pint-size jars, and keep refrigerated for up to 3 weeks.

A CLOSER LOOK: Cabbage is a humble ingredient that belongs to the cruciferous family and is packed with nutrients. This vegetable is high in vitamins B, C, and K as well as manganese, calcium, potassium, iron, magnesium, and phosphorus.

GINGERED ASPARAGUS

Serves 4 | Prep time: 10 minutes | Cook time: 12 minutes

Ginger adds a complexity of flavor and a healthy dose of antioxidants to this dish, creating a delicious side that fights inflammation. Ginger is very high in the antioxidants gingerol, shogaol, and paradol, which act similarly to NSAIDS (nonsteroidal anti-inflammatory drugs) to relieve pain. Gingerols can block the production of peroxynitrite, a free radical linked to inflammation and pain.

2 tablespoons grass-fed butter

2 teaspoons freshly grated ginger

Pinch ground nutmeg

24 asparagus spears, woody ends trimmed, halved

Himalayan salt or table salt, for seasoning

Freshly ground black pepper, for seasoning

1. In a large skillet over medium heat, melt the butter.
2. Add the ginger and nutmeg, and sauté for 2 minutes.
3. Add the asparagus and sauté for about 10 minutes, until just tender.
4. Season the asparagus with salt and pepper.

Per Serving: Calories: 87; Saturated Fat: 4g; Cholesterol: 15mg; Sodium: 103mg; Calcium: 30mg; Carbohydrates: 5g; Protein: 3g

BRAIN BOOSTER

GLUTEN-FREE

IMMUNE BOOSTER

NUT-FREE

PALEO-FRIENDLY

VEGETARIAN

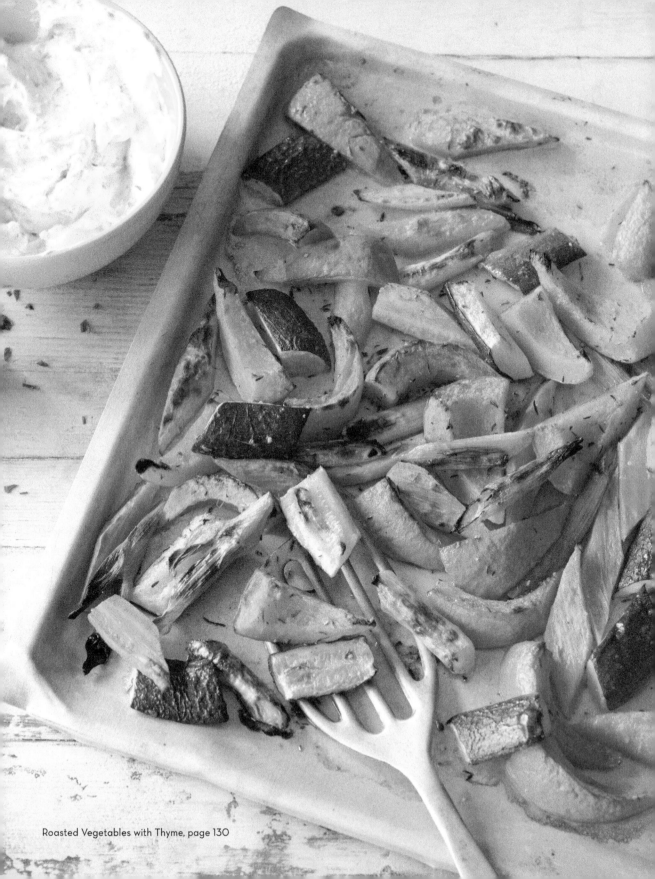

Roasted Vegetables with Thyme, page 130

8

vegetarian & vegan entrées

CHICKPEA BASIL-STUFFED
PEPPERS 124

ASPARAGUS WITH
SHALLOTS 125

SIMPLE FALAFEL 126

PORTOBELLO MUSHROOM-
BAKED EGGS 128

AVOCADO-CHICKPEA
TABBOULEH 129

ROASTED VEGETABLES
WITH THYME 130

CHOPPED VEGGIE

BOWL 131

SWEET POTATO AND
CHICKPEA SAUTÉ 132

CREAMY SUMMER
ZOODLES 134

WINTER VEGETABLE
STEW 135

CHICKPEA BASIL-STUFFED PEPPERS

Serves 4 | Prep time: 15 minutes | Cook time: 30 minutes

Many vegetables are used as handy containers for an assortment of delicious fillings. Bell peppers are popular because they are deep and bake up tender and sweet. This filling of chickpeas, tomatoes, cheese, olives, and basil has a Mediterranean flare that is very pleasing and packed with nutrients. These ingredients can help clear fibro fog, fight inflammation, and relieve the muscle pain associated with fibromyalgia.

4 red bell peppers, halved lengthwise
   and seeded
3 tablespoons extra-virgin olive oil
1 sweet onion, chopped
2 teaspoons minced garlic
1 cup sodium-free canned chickpeas, drained
1 cup halved cherry tomatoes
½ cup full-fat cottage cheese
½ cup chopped Kalamata olives
2 tablespoons chopped fresh basil leaves
Himalayan salt or table salt, for seasoning
Freshly ground black pepper, for seasoning

GLUTEN-FREE
IMMUNE BOOSTER
NUT-FREE
VEGETARIAN

1. Preheat the oven to 400°F.
2. Arrange the peppers, hollow-side up, on a rimmed baking sheet and set aside.
3. In a large skillet over medium-high heat, heat the olive oil.
4. Add the onion and garlic. Sauté for about 3 minutes, until softened.
5. Stir in the chickpeas, tomatoes, cottage cheese, olives, and basil. Cook for 5 minutes more.
6. Season the filling with salt and pepper, and spoon the filling into the peppers.
7. Bake for about 20 minutes, until the peppers are softened and the filling is heated through. Serve 2 halves per person.

Per Serving (2 stuffed halves): **Calories:** 267; Saturated Fat: 3g; Cholesterol: 2mg; Sodium: 332mg; Calcium: 160mg; Carbohydrates: 26g; Protein: 10g

ASPARAGUS WITH SHALLOTS

Serves 4 | Prep time: 20 minutes | Cook time: 15 minutes

Walnuts add a richness and delightful crunch to this simple dish. Walnuts contain alpha-linolenic acid, an essential omega-3 fatty acid that can help with mental clarity and combat fibro fog and stress. Oregano is also effective at clearing this symptom because it contains luteolin, a compound that helps reduce inflammation in the brain and preserve cognitive function. Luteolin increases the concentration of mood-boosting serotonin and dopamine, which reduce depression.

3 tablespoons extra-virgin olive oil

1 tablespoon grass-fed butter

1 leek, well cleaned and chopped

3 shallots, thinly sliced

2 teaspoons minced garlic

2 pounds asparagus, woody ends trimmed, cut into 2-inch pieces

2 cups cauliflower florets

Zest of 1 lemon

Juice of 1 lemon

¼ cup chopped walnuts

2 tablespoons chopped fresh oregano leaves

Himalayan salt or table salt, for seasoning

Freshly ground black pepper, for seasoning

1. In a large skillet over medium-high heat, heat the olive oil and melt the butter.
2. Add the leek, shallots, and garlic. Sauté for about 5 minutes, until tender.
3. Add the asparagus and cauliflower. Sauté for about 10 minutes more, until the vegetables are tender.
4. Stir in the lemon zest and juice, walnuts, and oregano.
5. Season the vegetables with salt and pepper and serve.

Per Serving: Calories: 232; Saturated Fat: 5g; Cholesterol: 8mg; Sodium: 105mg; Calcium: 90mg; Carbohydrates: 17g; Protein: 7g

BRAIN BOOSTER

GLUTEN-FREE

IMMUNE BOOSTER

PALEO-FRIENDLY

VEGETARIAN

SIMPLE FALAFEL

Serves 4 | Prep time: 15 minutes | Cook time: 16 minutes

Falafel is a traditional Middle Eastern food usually made with a combination of chickpeas and fava beans. This version uses only chickpeas to conform to the fibromyalgia diet, which prohibits legumes and also excludes the pita pocket for its gluten. The main ingredients here—those chickpeas, along with kale, almonds, and tahini—are packed with antioxidants, vitamins, minerals, healthy fats, and protein. Falafel has a very beneficial fat/protein/carbohydrate ratio and can be part of a balanced diet for people with fibromyalgia.

1 (16-ounce) can water-packed
   chickpeas, drained

4 cups chopped kale

¼ cup almond flour, plus more as needed

4 garlic cloves, lightly crushed

2 tablespoons tahini

Juice of ½ lemon, plus more as needed

½ teaspoon ground cumin

Pinch Himalayan salt or table salt

¼ cup extra-virgin olive oil

BRAIN BOOSTER
DAIRY-FREE
GLUTEN-FREE
IMMUNE BOOSTER
VEGETARIAN

1. In a food processor, combine the chickpeas, kale, almond flour, garlic, tahini, lemon juice, cumin, and salt. Pulse until the mixture holds together when pressed. If the mixture is too dry, add more lemon juice, a little at a time; if too wet, add more almond flour, a little at a time.

2. Roll the falafel mixture into golf ball–size disks, flatten them to about ½ inch thick, and place them on a plate in the refrigerator until firm.

3. In a large skillet over medium-high heat, heat the olive oil.

4. Arrange the falafel in the skillet, do not overcrowd, and panfry them for about 8 minutes, turning once halfway through, until golden on both sides. Transfer to paper towels to drain.

5. Repeat with the remaining falafel.

6. Serve immediately. Refrigerate leftovers in an airtight container for 3 days, or freeze for up to 1 month.

Per Serving: **Calories: 267; Saturated Fat: 3g; Cholesterol: 0mg; Sodium: 103mg; Calcium: 200mg; Carbohydrates: 16g; Protein: 8g**

A CLOSER LOOK: Tahini adds a nutty, rich taste to the falafel. Tahini is made from ground sesame seeds and is a stellar source of vitamins B_1, B_2, and E, as well as calcium and magnesium.

PORTOBELLO MUSHROOM-
BAKED EGGS

Serves 4 | Prep time: 15 minutes | Cook time: 22 minutes

Mushrooms are the only vegetable that contains vitamin D in the form of a plant sterol called ergosterol, the precursor of vitamin D₂. Vitamin D is crucial for easing muscle pain.

8 large portobello mushrooms, stemmed,
   black gills scooped out
¼ cup extra-virgin olive oil, divided
¼ sweet onion, chopped
1 teaspoon minced garlic
2 cups chopped fresh spinach
1 sweet potato, shredded
Himalayan salt or table salt, for seasoning
Freshly ground black pepper, for seasoning
8 eggs
¼ teaspoon paprika
1 tablespoon chopped fresh parsley leaves

BRAIN BOOSTER
DAIRY-FREE
GLUTEN-FREE
IMMUNE BOOSTER
NUT-FREE
PALEO-FRIENDLY
VEGETARIAN

Per Serving (2 stuffed mushrooms): **Calories:** 310;
Saturated Fat: 6g; Cholesterol: 327mg; Sodium: 205mg;
Calcium: 70mg; Carbohydrates: 10g; Protein: 14g

1. Preheat the oven to 400°F.
2. Line a rimmed baking sheet with parchment paper.
3. Rub the mushrooms all over with 4 teaspoons olive oil, and place them, hollow-side down, on the prepared sheet.
4. Bake for about 5 minutes, until softened. Remove from the oven and flip.
5. While the mushrooms bake, in a large skillet over medium-high heat, heat the remaining 2 tablespoons plus 2 teaspoons olive oil.
6. Add the onion and garlic. Sauté for about 2 minutes, until softened.
7. Stir in the spinach and sweet potato. Cook for about 5 minutes, until softened.
8. Season the filling with salt and pepper, and divide it among the mushrooms, pressing it into the hollows.
9. Crack 1 egg over each filled mushroom.
10. Bake the mushrooms for about 10 minutes, until the eggs set. Serve.

AVOCADO-CHICKPEA TABBOULEH

Serves 4 | Prep time: 30 minutes | Cook time: 0 minutes

Tabbouleh is usually made with grains or couscous, but the chopped cauliflower and chickpeas provide an equally satisfying base for this dish. Mint and parsley, traditional in tabbouleh, are also included in this version because they taste fabulous and offer health benefits. Mint contains melatonin, an important sleep hormone that can help alleviate sleep issues such as insomnia or sleep apnea.

2 (16-ounce) cans water-packed
   chickpeas, drained
2 cups finely chopped cauliflower
2 cups halved cherry tomatoes
1 English cucumber, chopped
1 avocado, peeled, pitted, and diced
2 scallions, white and green parts, chopped
Zest of 1 lemon
Juice of 1 lemon
½ cup chopped fresh parsley leaves
¼ cup chopped fresh mint leaves
¼ cup extra-virgin olive oil
Himalayan salt or table salt, for seasoning
Freshly ground black pepper, for seasoning

1. In a large bowl, stir together the chickpeas, cauliflower, tomatoes, cucumber, avocado, scallions, lemon zest and juice, parsley, mint, and olive oil.
2. Season the tabbouleh with salt and pepper. Serve.

Per Serving: Calories: 294; Saturated Fat: 4g; Cholesterol: 0mg; Sodium: 93mg; Calcium: 120mg; Carbohydrates: 2g; Protein: 7g

BRAIN BOOSTER
DAIRY-FREE
GLUTEN-FREE
IMMUNE BOOSTER
NUT-FREE
VEGETARIAN

ROASTED VEGETABLES WITH THYME

Serves 4 | Prep time: 10 minutes | Cook time: 45 minutes

The scent of roasting vegetables caramelizing in the oven will waft through the house like a dinner bell. Squash and carrots are wonderful sources of beta-carotene; zucchini is high in vitamin A and potassium; olive oil is a healthy monounsaturated fat. This combination of ingredients can reduce inflammation and ensure there is good blood flow to muscles so they can function effectively. Change the types of vegetables in this dish depending on your preference.

1 butternut squash, peeled, halved, pulp and seeds removed, cut into thick strips

2 carrots, cut into chunks

2 zucchini, cut into chunks

2 scallions, white and green parts, cut into 2-inch pieces

3 tablespoons extra-virgin olive oil

2 teaspoons chopped fresh thyme leaves

Himalayan salt or table salt, for seasoning

Freshly ground black pepper, for seasoning

BRAIN BOOSTER
DAIRY-FREE
GLUTEN-FREE
IMMUNE BOOSTER
NUT-FREE
PALEO-FRIENDLY
VEGETARIAN

1. Preheat the oven to 400°F.
2. Line a rimmed baking sheet with aluminum foil.
3. In a large bowl toss together the squash, carrots, zucchini, scallions, olive oil, and thyme. Transfer the vegetables to the prepared sheet.
4. Bake for about 45 minutes, until they are tender and lightly browned, stirring occasionally.
5. Season with salt and pepper and serve.

Per Serving: Calories: 202; Saturated Fat: 2g; Cholesterol: 0mg; Sodium: 78mg; Calcium: 124mg; Carbohydrates: 28g; Protein: 4g

CHOPPED VEGGIE BOWL

Serves 4 | Prep time: 25 minutes | Cook time: 16 minutes

"Bowls" are an ever-expanding culinary trend found in home kitchens as well as casual and fine-dining establishments. They combine an assortment of ingredients, herbs, meats (in some cases), and tasty sauces in one convenient single-serving bowl. The various colors of the plentiful vegetables in this recipe highlight the broad range of antioxidants available in this dish to combat inflammation. The olive oil, sunflower seeds, and hazelnuts contain omega-3 fatty acids and tryptophan to support brain health and help you sleep better.

3 tablespoons extra-virgin olive oil

1 sweet onion, chopped

2 teaspoons minced garlic

1 teaspoon grated fresh ginger

2 cups roughly chopped cauliflower

2 cups chopped broccoli

2 cups shredded red cabbage

2 celery stalks, chopped

2 carrots, shredded

1 cup chopped Swiss chard

2 tablespoons balsamic vinegar

1 teaspoon ground cumin

½ teaspoon ground coriander

½ cup sunflower seeds

¼ cup chopped toasted hazelnuts

1. In a large skillet over medium-high heat, heat the olive oil.
2. Add the onion, garlic, and ginger. Sauté for about 3 minutes, until softened.
3. Stir in the cauliflower, broccoli, red cabbage, celery, and carrots. Sauté for about 10 minutes, until the vegetables are crisp-tender.
4. Stir in the chard, balsamic vinegar, cumin, and coriander. Sauté for about 3 minutes, until the chard is wilted.
5. Sprinkle with the sunflower seeds and hazelnuts. Serve.

SIMPLIFY IT: A food processor can be used to do all the chopping for this recipe if you want the job done quickly and efficiently. Just put in a shredding or slicing disk, and cut everything in the processor bowl.

Per Serving: Calories: 224; Saturated Fat: 3g; Cholesterol: 0mg; Sodium: 87mg; Calcium: 90mg; Carbohydrates: 17g; Protein: 7g

BRAIN BOOSTER
DAIRY-FREE
GLUTEN-FREE
IMMUNE BOOSTER
PALEO-FRIENDLY
VEGETARIAN

SWEET POTATO AND CHICKPEA SAUTÉ

Serves 4 | Prep time: 20 minutes | Cook time: 25 minutes

Simple and filling is often all you need to end a tiring day or enjoy as a light lunch when you have a stressful or activity-packed morning or afternoon. If you've ever thought vegetarian meals to be insubstantial, this root vegetable and chickpea creation will certainly change your mind. You may feel an increase in energy (but without a spike in blood sugar), a sharpening of concentration, and a welcome lessening of anxiety after eating a heaping bowl of this sauté.

BRAIN BOOSTER
DAIRY-FREE
GLUTEN-FREE
IMMUNE BOOSTER
NUT-FREE
VEGETARIAN

For the dressing

¼ cup extra-virgin olive oil

2 tablespoons apple cider vinegar

1 teaspoon xylitol

½ teaspoon ground cinnamon

Himalayan salt or table salt, for seasoning

Freshly ground black pepper, for seasoning

For the veggies

3 sweet potatoes, diced

1 celeriac, peeled and diced

1 carrot, diced

1 parsnip, diced

1 tablespoon extra-virgin olive oil

1 (16-ounce) can water-packed chickpeas, drained

1 scallion, white and green parts, sliced

½ cup pumpkin seeds

To make the dressing

1. In a small bowl, whisk the olive oil, cider vinegar, xylitol, and cinnamon until well blended.
2. Season with salt and pepper. Set aside.

To make the salad

1. Preheat the oven to 350°F.
2. Line a rimmed baking sheet with parchment paper.
3. In a large bowl, toss together the sweet potatoes, celeriac, carrot, parsnip, and olive oil until well coated. Spread the vegetables on the prepared sheet.
4. Bake for about 25 minutes, until tender and lightly caramelized.
5. Remove the vegetables from the oven, and let them cool for 15 minutes.
6. Transfer the roasted vegetables to a large bowl, and toss them with the dressing, chickpeas, and scallion.
7. Serve topped with pumpkin seeds.

COOKING TIP: This dish is very versatile and can be served either hot or cold. Toss the vegetables with the dressing while still warm from the oven so it soaks in. Serve the dish immediately, or chill the dish for a later time.

Per Serving: Calories: 485; Saturated Fat: 4g; Cholesterol: 0mg; Sodium: 169mg; Calcium: 113mg; Carbohydrates: 59g; Protein: 10g

CREAMY SUMMER ZOODLES

Serves 4 | Prep time: 20 minutes | Cook time: 0 minutes

This dish is a study in glorious greens: pale avocado, creamy white and green zucchini noodles, bright edamame, and dark green kale. It is stunning and crammed with vitamins B₁₂, C, and D as well as folic acid and magnesium. Sleep issues, fatigue, fibro fog, and pain are all addressed with this combination of nutrients, which means it is a beneficial choice for a light lunch or snack.

For the sauce

2 avocados, peeled and pitted

½ cup heavy (whipping) cream

Juice of 1 lime

2 tablespoons chopped fresh cilantro leaves

1 teaspoon xylitol

1 teaspoon ground cumin

¼ teaspoon ground coriander

Pinch Himalayan salt or table salt

For the zoodles

4 zucchini, spiralized or julienned

2 cups edamame

1 cup shredded kale

To make the sauce

In a blender, combine the avocados, heavy cream, lime juice, cilantro, xylitol, cumin, coriander, and salt. Pulse until smooth. Set aside.

To make the zoodles

1. In a large bowl, toss together the zucchini, edamame, and kale.
2. Add the dressing and toss to coat. Serve.

Per Serving: Calories: 464; Saturated Fat: 8g; Cholesterol: 21mg; Sodium: 103mg; Calcium: 310mg; Carbohydrates: 26g; Protein: 21g

BRAIN BOOSTER
GLUTEN-FREE
IMMUNE BOOSTER
NUT-FREE
VEGETARIAN

WINTER VEGETABLE STEW

Serves 4 | Prep time: 25 minutes | Cook time: 40 minutes

The vegetables in this stew are sautéed in coconut oil. Coconut oil used to be considered an ingredient to avoid because it is a saturated fat, but recent recommendations show it has many health benefits and produces none of the problems that come from ingesting excess animal-based saturated fats. Coconut oil is a good choice for a fibromyalgia diet because it can balance hormones, decrease joint pain, and improve memory and cognitive function.

3 tablespoons coconut oil

1 sweet onion, chopped

2 teaspoons minced garlic

2 sweet potatoes, diced

2 carrots, diced

2 parsnips, diced

1 celeriac, peeled and diced

6 cups gluten-free, sodium-free
   vegetable broth

1 tablespoon chopped fresh basil leaves

1 teaspoon chopped fresh oregano leaves

2 tomatoes, diced

2 cups shredded fresh spinach

½ cup heavy (whipping) cream

Himalayan salt or table salt, for seasoning

Freshly ground black pepper, for seasoning

1. In a large saucepan over medium-high heat, heat the coconut oil.
2. Add the onion and garlic. Sauté for about 3 minutes, until softened.
3. Add the sweet potatoes, carrots, parsnips, celeriac, vegetable broth, basil, and oregano. Bring to a boil, reduce the heat to low, and simmer for about 30 minutes until the vegetables are tender.
4. Stir in the tomatoes, spinach, and heavy cream. Simmer for 5 minutes more.
5. Season the stew with salt and pepper. Serve.

Per Serving: Calories: 396; Saturated Fat: 10g; Cholesterol: 21mg; Sodium: 196mg; Calcium: 134mg; Carbohydrates: 57g; Protein: 7g

BRAIN BOOSTER
GLUTEN-FREE
IMMUNE BOOSTER
VEGETARIAN

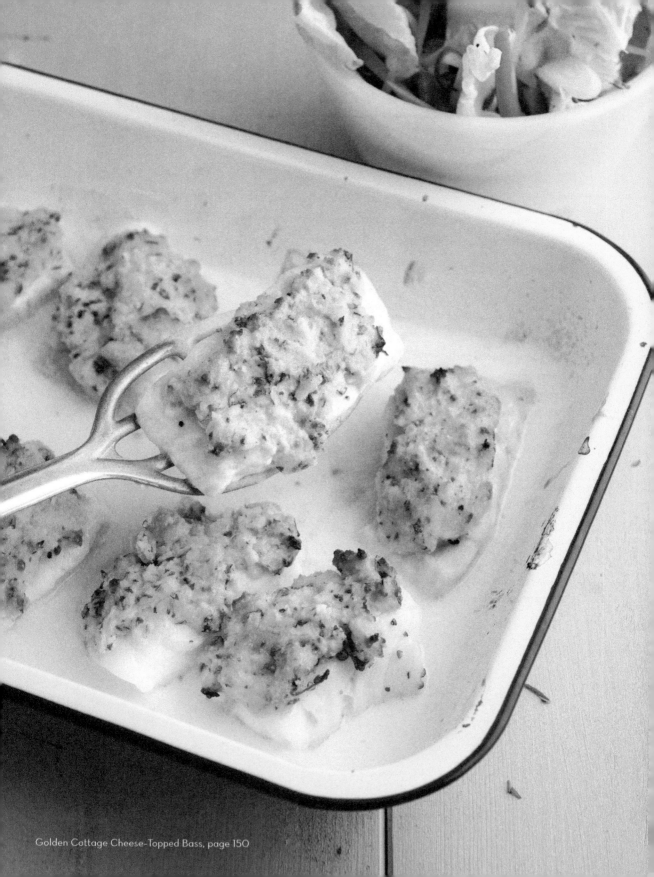

Golden Cottage Cheese-Topped Bass, page 150

9
fish & seafood entrées

MUSSELS IN COCONUT
BROTH 138

CAJUN SCALLOPS 139

GARLIC SHRIMP AND
VEGETABLES 140

TROUT-PUMPKIN
PATTIES 141

SHRIMP EGG
FOO YOUNG 142

GREEK FISH STEW 144

ROASTED SOLE WITH
VEGETABLES, GARLIC,
AND SUNFLOWER
SEEDS 146

ORANGE-PISTACHIO
BASS 147

COCONUT-TOMATO
SEAFOOD CURRY 148

GOLDEN COTTAGE
CHEESE-TOPPED BASS 150

HARISSA-RUBBED
BASS 151

PANFRIED TILAPIA WITH
COMPOUND BUTTER 152

SPICE-RUBBED FLOUNDER
WITH CITRUS SALSA 154

COCONUT MILK-BAKED
CATFISH 156

ROASTED TROUT
WITH FENNEL 157

BAKED SOLE WITH
PARSLEY PISTOU 158

TOMATO-BAKED BASS 159

ROASTED BELL
PEPPER TROUT 160

SOLE WITH GINGER-WASABI
GLAZE 162

BAKED TILAPIA WITH
BLUEBERRY-AVOCADO
SALSA 163

MUSSELS IN COCONUT BROTH

Serves 4 | Prep time: 20 minutes | Cook time: 13 minutes

Mussels are underused in home kitchens because they look like a great deal of work. They aren't—all you have to do is scrub them, pull out the long hair-like beard, and discard any that are open. Mussels are high in vitamins B$_{12}$ and C to reduce muscle aches and inflammation, omega-3 fatty acids to reduce inflammation, protein to rebuild damaged cells, and magnesium to decrease stiffness and joint pain.

1 tablespoon extra-virgin olive oil

2 teaspoons minced garlic

1 teaspoon grated fresh ginger

½ cup coconut milk

½ cup gluten-free, sodium-free chicken broth

Zest of 1 lemon

Juice of 1 lemon

1 tablespoon chopped fresh basil leaves

1½ pounds fresh mussels, scrubbed
    and debearded

Freshly ground black pepper, for seasoning

1 scallion, white and green parts, thinly
    sliced on a bias

1. In a large skillet over medium-high heat, heat the olive oil.
2. Add the garlic and ginger. Sauté for about 3 minutes, until softened.
3. Stir in the coconut milk, chicken broth, lemon zest and juice, and basil. Bring the mixture to a boil.
4. Add the mussels to the skillet, cover, and steam the mussels for about 10 minutes, until the shells open. Remove the skillet from the heat, and discard any unopened shells.
5. Season the mussels with pepper, and stir in the scallion. Serve.

Per Serving: Calories: 254; Saturated Fat: 6g; Cholesterol: 48mg; Sodium: 435mg; Calcium: 63mg; Carbohydrates: 9g; Protein: 21g

BRAIN BOOSTER
DAIRY-FREE
GLUTEN-FREE
IMMUNE BOOSTER
PALEO-FRIENDLY

CAJUN SCALLOPS

Serves 4 | Prep time: 15 minutes | Cook time: 11 minutes

Scallops are mild, tender-fleshed mollusks that soak up flavors well, so spices and herbs have a tremendous impact. Scallops, like most seafood, are an excellent source of an amino acid called L-carnitine, which can help reduce muscle pain and depression. Scallops are also rich in vitamin B_{12} and omega-3 fatty acids, crucial nutrients for boosting energy and fighting inflammation.

1 teaspoon garlic powder

1 teaspoon paprika

½ teaspoon Himalayan salt or table salt

½ teaspoon dried oregano

½ teaspoon freshly ground black pepper

½ teaspoon onion powder

½ teaspoon cayenne pepper

3 tablespoons extra-virgin olive oil

1 sweet onion, thinly sliced

1 teaspoon minced garlic

1 teaspoon grass-fed butter

1 pound fresh scallops, cleaned

BRAIN BOOSTER
GLUTEN-FREE
IMMUNE BOOSTER
NUT-FREE
PALEO-FRIENDLY

Per Serving: Calories: 168; Saturated Fat: 3g; Cholesterol: 40mg; Sodium: 264mg; Calcium: 30mg; Carbohydrates: 3g; Protein: 20g

1. In a small bowl, stir together the garlic powder, paprika, salt, oregano, pepper, onion powder, and cayenne until well blended.
2. In a large skillet over medium-high heat, heat the olive oil.
3. Add the onion, garlic, and spice blend. Sauté for about 3 minutes, until the onion softens.
4. Move the vegetables to the side of the skillet, and add the butter to melt.
5. Arrange the scallops in the skillet in a single layer, and panfry for 4 minutes. Flip and cook for about 4 minutes more, until just cooked through and tender.
6. Stir the vegetables back into the scallops and serve.

SIMPLIFY IT: The spice blend, or Cajun seasoning, can be mixed up ahead and kept in a small sealed container at room temperature for up to 1 month. Use a premade Cajun seasoning if you have a brand you enjoy.

GARLIC SHRIMP
AND VEGETABLES

Serves 4 | Prep time: 20 minutes | Cook time: 12 minutes

This versatile dish that cooks in one skillet with heaps of colorful vegetables and tender sautéed shrimp can serve as a main course as well as a side dish. Shrimp is a stellar source of the antioxidant carotenoid, astaxanthin. This antioxidant supports and protects both the nervous system and musculoskeletal system.

3 tablespoons grass-fed butter

1 red bell pepper, diced

1 yellow bell pepper, diced

1 pound asparagus, woody ends trimmed,
   cut into 1-inch pieces

2 cups cauliflower florets

2 teaspoons minced garlic

Zest of 1 lemon

¼ teaspoon Himalayan salt or table salt

⅛ teaspoon freshly ground black pepper

1 tablespoon extra-virgin olive oil

1 pound raw shrimp (26 to 30 count),
   peeled and deveined

1 cup gluten-free, sodium-free chicken broth

1 teaspoon arrowroot powder

Juice of 1 lemon

1 scallion, white and green parts, chopped

1. In a large skillet over medium-high heat, melt the butter.
2. Add the red and yellow bell peppers, asparagus, cauliflower, garlic, and lemon zest. Sauté for about 6 minutes, until the vegetables are tender. Transfer the vegetables to a bowl, season with salt and pepper, and set aside.
3. Return the skillet to the heat. Add the olive oil and shrimp. Sauté for 1 minute.
4. In a small bowl, whisk the broth and arrowroot powder. Pour this mixture into the skillet. Cook for about 5 minutes, stirring constantly, until the sauce thickens and the shrimp are cooked through.
5. Stir in the vegetables, lemon juice, and scallion. Serve.

Per Serving: Calories: 308; Saturated Fat: 5g; Cholesterol: 246mg; Sodium: 434mg; Calcium: 154mg; Carbohydrates: 14g; Protein: 30g

BRAIN BOOSTER
GLUTEN-FREE
IMMUNE BOOSTER
NUT-FREE
PALEO-FRIENDLY

TROUT-PUMPKIN PATTIES

Serves 4 | Prep time: 20 minutes | Cook time: 15 minutes

Fish sticks and cakes gained a very bad reputation in the 1970s and '80s because they were packed with preservatives and tasted awful. This golden fish patty has a great deal of flavor from capsaicin-rich red pepper flakes and antioxidant-packed garlic. The almond flour and eggs are binding ingredients that also provide cell-building protein and inflammation-fighting fats. Substitute sweet potato or squash if pumpkin is not available.

1 pound pumpkin, cooked and mashed

12 ounces cooked trout, flaked

½ cup almond flour

2 eggs

¼ sweet onion, chopped

½ red bell pepper, chopped

1 scallion, white and green parts, chopped

1 teaspoon minced garlic

Pinch red pepper flakes

Pinch Himalayan salt or table salt

3 tablespoons extra-virgin olive oil

BRAIN BOOSTER
DAIRY-FREE
GLUTEN-FREE
IMMUNE BOOSTER
PALEO-FRIENDLY

1. Preheat the oven to 400°F.
2. Line a rimmed baking sheet with parchment paper and set aside.
3. In a large bowl, stir together the pumpkin, trout, almond flour, eggs, onion, red bell pepper, scallion, garlic, red pepper flakes, and salt until well mixed. Shape the mixture into 8 patties, about ½ inch thick.
4. Arrange the patties on the prepared sheet, and brush both sides of each patty with the olive oil.
5. Bake for about 15 minutes, turning once halfway through, until the patties are golden brown.

SIMPLIFY IT: Baking or blanching fresh pumpkin is not difficult, but you might end up with much more than you need, depending on the size of the squash. To save time, use 1 can of 100 percent pure pumpkin with no added sugar for this recipe instead.

Per Serving: Calories: 241; Saturated Fat: 4g; Cholesterol: 145mg; Sodium: 156mg; Calcium: 114mg; Carbohydrates: 13g; Protein: 29g

SHRIMP EGG FOO YOUNG

Serves 2 | Prep time: 15 minutes | Cook time: 25 minutes

Egg foo young is really just a fancy omelet, with a great deal of vegetables and shrimp in this variation. The fibromyalgia diet usually avoids legumes, but the sprouts used in this dish are considered a healthy compromise. Soaking and sprouting legumes removes the enzyme inhibitor, which in turn promotes retention of minerals and better digestion. Bean sprouts are high in fiber, vitamins A, B-complex, C, and E as well as essential fatty acids.

1 tablespoon extra-virgin olive oil

1 teaspoon sesame oil

2 teaspoons minced garlic

1 teaspoon grated fresh ginger

½ pound raw shrimp (26 to 30 count), peeled and deveined

2 cups bean sprouts

2 scallions, white and green parts, chopped

6 eggs

¼ teaspoon Himalayan salt or table salt

BRAIN BOOSTER
DAIRY-FREE
GLUTEN-FREE
IMMUNE BOOSTER
NUT-FREE
PALEO-FRIENDLY

1. In a large skillet or wok over medium heat, heat the olive oil and sesame oil.
2. Add the garlic and ginger. Sauté for about 3 minutes, until softened.
3. Add the shrimp. Sauté for about 6 minutes, until pink and cooked through.
4. Stir in the bean sprouts and scallions. Sauté for 5 minutes, spreading the vegetables and shrimp out in the skillet.
5. In a small bowl, beat together the eggs and salt. Pour the eggs into the skillet, and gently use the edge of your cooking utensil to make spaces in the veggies and shrimp for the eggs to seep through to the skillet's surface. Cook for about 5 minutes until the eggs are set on the bottom.

6. Cut the omelet into quarters, and flip each over. Cook for about 5 minutes more, until the omelet is completely cooked through.

7. Serve 2 pieces per person.

Per Serving (2 pieces): **Calories:** 468; **Saturated Fat:** 6g; **Cholesterol:** 634mg; **Sodium:** 678mg; **Calcium:** 214mg; **Carbohydrates:** 14g; **Protein:** 50g

COOKING TIP: Peeling and deveining shrimp is not difficult, but it can be messy and take some time. Buy already cleaned shrimp, or even cooked shrimp, for your recipe needs.

GREEK FISH STEW

Serves 4 | Prep time: 20 minutes | Cook time: 20 minutes

There is something comforting about a steaming bowl of stew studded with pale pink shrimp, pretty mussels, and chunks of protein-rich fish. All the flavors you might enjoy in a sunny Mediterranean country are present in this stew: tomatoes, rich black olives, artichokes, and iron-packed spinach. The diet from this part of the world is often recommended for fibromites because it includes unprocessed foods, full-fat dairy, olive oil, and good-quality proteins and seafood.

BRAIN BOOSTER
DAIRY-FREE
GLUTEN-FREE
IMMUNE BOOSTER
NUT-FREE
PALEO-FRIENDLY

3 tablespoons extra-virgin olive oil

1 sweet onion, diced

2 teaspoons minced garlic

2 red bell peppers, diced

1 cup quartered water-packed, canned artichoke hearts

1 (28-ounce) can sodium-free diced tomatoes

1 cup gluten-free, sodium-free fish broth

Zest of 1 lemon

Juice of 1 lemon

1 pound whitefish fillet, cut into chunks

½ pound shrimp, peeled and deveined

½ pound mussels, scrubbed and debearded

1 cup shredded fresh spinach

½ cup sliced Kalamata olives

¼ cup chopped fresh parsley leaves

Himalayan salt or table salt, for seasoning

Freshly ground black pepper, for seasoning

1. In a large stockpot over medium-high heat, heat the olive oil.
2. Add the onion and garlic. Sauté for about 3 minutes, until translucent.
3. Add the red bell peppers and artichoke hearts. Sauté for about 3 minutes.
4. Stir in the tomatoes, fish broth, lemon zest, and juice, and bring the mixture to a boil.
5. Stir in the fish, shrimp, and mussels. Cover the pot, reduce the heat to low, and simmer for about 10 minutes until the mussels open. Remove and discard any unopened mussels.
6. Stir in the spinach, olives, and parsley. Simmer for 1 minute more and remove from the heat.
7. Season with salt and pepper. Serve.

Per Serving: Calories: 416; Saturated Fat: 3g; Cholesterol: 135mg; Sodium: 564mg; Calcium: 154mg; Carbohydrates: 24g; Protein: 45g

ROASTED SOLE WITH VEGETABLES, GARLIC, AND SUNFLOWER SEEDS

Serves 4 | Prep time: 20 minutes | Cook time: 40 minutes

This colorful dish, with vibrant beets and earthy Swiss chard, gives you a double dose of naturally occurring sodium. Though you may think sodium is not a healthy mineral—likely due to the many warnings about hypertension or other conditions exacerbated by consuming too much—sodium has been linked with reducing the fatigue, insomnia, and pain levels in people with fibromyalgia.

6 beets, peeled and halved

3 carrots, cut into 2-inch chunks

3 parsnips, cut into 2-inch chunks

1 red onion, cut into eight wedges

6 garlic cloves, quartered

3 tablespoons extra-virgin olive oil, divided

Himalayan salt or table salt, for seasoning

Freshly ground black pepper, for seasoning

3 cups (2-inch pieces) deribbed Swiss chard

4 (6-ounce) sole fillets

1 tablespoon freshly squeezed lemon juice

½ cup sunflower seeds

BRAIN BOOSTER

DAIRY-FREE

GLUTEN-FREE

IMMUNE BOOSTER

NUT-FREE

PALEO-FRIENDLY

1. Preheat the oven to 400°F.
2. On a rimmed baking sheet, arrange the beets, carrots, parsnips, red onion, and garlic. Drizzle the vegetables with 2 tablespoons olive oil. Season with salt and pepper.
3. Roast the vegetables for 30 minutes, turning several times.
4. Stir in the Swiss chard, and move the veggies to clear about one-fourth of the baking sheet for the fish.
5. Arrange the fish in the empty space on the sheet. Drizzle it with lemon juice and the remaining tablespoon olive oil.
6. Roast the fish and vegetables for about 10 minutes, until the fish is just cooked through and the vegetables are tender.
7. Serve topped with sunflower seeds.

Per Serving: Calories: 503; Saturated Fat: 3g; Cholesterol: 116mg; Sodium: 445mg; Calcium: 141mg; Carbohydrates: 42g; Protein: 48g

ORANGE-PISTACHIO BASS

Serves 4 | Prep time: 15 minutes | Cook time: 21 minutes

Orange sauce might seem more at home on duck or chicken, but it is equally delicious on flaky white bass. Oranges are high in vitamin C, fiber, B vitamins, calcium, and a wide range of phytonutrients. Many of the inflammation-fighting phytonutrients are in the peel, so make sure you zest it before peeling and segmenting the orange.

4 (5-ounce) bass fillets

Himalayan salt or table salt, for seasoning

Freshly ground black pepper, for seasoning

2 tablespoons extra-virgin olive oil

1 tablespoon grass-fed butter

2 shallots, minced

2 tablespoons apple cider vinegar

2 oranges, peeled, segmented,
    and roughly chopped

¼ cup freshly squeezed orange juice

1 tablespoon grated orange zest

¼ cup chopped pistachios

2 tablespoons chopped fresh oregano leaves

BRAIN BOOSTER
GLUTEN-FREE
IMMUNE BOOSTER
PALEO-FRIENDLY

1. Pat the fish dry with paper towels, and lightly season with salt and pepper.
2. In a large skillet over medium-high heat, heat the olive oil.
3. Add the fish and cook for about 18 minutes, turning once halfway through, until the fillets are opaque and cooked through. Transfer the fish to a plate, and cover with aluminum foil to keep warm.
4. Return the skillet to the heat. Add the butter to melt.
5. Add the shallots. Sauté for about 1 minute, until softened.
6. Stir in the cider vinegar, oranges, orange juice, and orange zest. Bring the mixture to a boil, reduce the heat to low, and simmer for 2 minutes.
7. Stir in the pistachios, and serve the fish with a scoop of orange sauce sprinkled with oregano.

Per Serving: Calories: 372; Saturated Fat: 6g; Cholesterol: 131mg; Sodium: 228mg; Calcium: 235mg; Carbohydrates: 16g; Protein: 36g

COCONUT-TOMATO
SEAFOOD CURRY

Serves 6 | Prep time: 20 minutes | Cook time: 30 minutes

This curry does not conform to any particular traditional curry dish but instead contains elements of several, such as rogan josh and madras. The addition of tomatoes and creamy coconut milk places this dish in its own category. Red curry paste comes in mild, medium, or hot versions, so make your choice to suit your palate. Keep in mind that the hotter the spice paste, the more capsaicin is in it, and capsaicin can help relieve the pain associated with fibromyalgia.

BRAIN BOOSTER
DAIRY-FREE
GLUTEN-FREE
IMMUNE BOOSTER
PALEO-FRIENDLY

1 tablespoon extra-virgin olive oil

1 sweet onion, chopped

1 red bell pepper, diced

1 carrot, diced

1 tablespoon minced garlic

1 tablespoon grated fresh ginger

3 cups coconut milk

1 cup gluten-free, sodium-free chicken broth

2 tomatoes, diced

2 tablespoons red curry paste

1 pound whitefish fillet (any firm fish allowed in the diet)

1 pound shrimp, peeled, deveined, and roughly chopped

2 cups cauliflower florets

2 cups quartered baby bok choy

1 cup shredded kale

Himalayan salt or table salt, for seasoning

Freshly ground black pepper, for seasoning

¼ cup slivered almonds

1. In a large saucepan over medium heat, heat the olive oil.
2. Add the onion, red bell pepper, carrot, garlic, and ginger. Sauté for about 10 minutes until softened.
3. Stir in the coconut milk, chicken broth, tomatoes, and curry paste. Increase the heat to high, and bring the mixture to a boil.
4. Reduce the heat to medium. Add the fish, shrimp, cauliflower, and bok choy. Simmer for about 10 minutes, until the seafood is cooked through.
5. Stir in the kale and season with salt and pepper. Simmer for about 5 minutes more, until the kale is wilted.
6. Serve topped with the almonds.

Per Serving: Calories: 650; Saturated Fat: 27g; Cholesterol: 185mg; Sodium: 764mg; Calcium: 163mg; Carbohydrates: 31g; Protein: 35g

A CLOSER LOOK: Curry is not a single spice but a complex combination of many different ingredients, such as turmeric, cumin, coriander, paprika, ginger, and cloves. Mix your own creation rather than using curry paste if you enjoy certain spices more than others.

GOLDEN COTTAGE CHEESE-TOPPED BASS

Serves 4 | Prep time: 20 minutes | Cook time: 20 minutes

Cheese and fish might seem like a strange combination until you recall that delectable creamy seafood lasagna made with cottage cheese is extremely popular. The cheese topping keeps the fish moist and adds healthy fats and B-complex vitamins as well as calcium and magnesium. This is a potent anti-inflammatory pain-relieving combination to add to the protein in the fish.

4 (6-ounce) bass fillets, washed and patted dry

Himalayan salt or table salt, for seasoning

Freshly ground black pepper, for seasoning

1 cup full-fat cottage cheese

¼ cup almond flour

1 teaspoon minced garlic

1 tablespoon chopped fresh basil leaves

Lemon slices, for serving

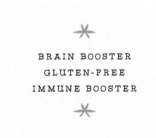

BRAIN BOOSTER

GLUTEN-FREE

IMMUNE BOOSTER

1. Preheat the oven to 375°F.
2. Lightly season the fillets with salt and pepper, and place them in a 9-by-9-inch baking dish.
3. In a small bowl, stir together the cottage cheese, almond flour, garlic, and basil until well mixed. Spread the cheese mixture evenly over the fish.
4. Bake the fish for about 20 minutes, until it is just cooked through and the topping is bubbly and golden.
5. Serve with the lemon slices.

Per Serving: Calories: 386; Saturated Fat: 4g; Cholesterol: 5mg; Sodium: 271mg; Calcium: 64mg; Carbohydrates: 4g; Protein: 47g

HARISSA-RUBBED BASS

Serves 4 | Prep time: 15 minutes | Cook time: 35 minutes

The bright color of harissa is an indicator that this spread is bursting with inflammation-fighting antioxidants such as beta-carotene. Harissa is also a wonderful choice for other proteins like poultry, lamb, and pork, so make sure you make extra. Add a little heat to the harissa with a pinch of red pepper flakes. This addition will also add pain-relieving capsaicin.

1 red bell pepper

½ cup oil-packed sun-dried tomatoes

3 garlic cloves

3 tablespoons extra-virgin olive oil

2 tablespoons freshly squeezed lemon juice

1 teaspoon ground cumin

1 teaspoon ground coriander

½ teaspoon caraway seeds

¼ teaspoon Himalayan salt or table salt

4 (6-ounce) bass fillets

BRAIN BOOSTER
DAIRY-FREE
GLUTEN-FREE
IMMUNE BOOSTER
NUT-FREE
PALEO-FRIENDLY

Per Serving: Calories: 373; Saturated Fat: 4g; Cholesterol: 148mg; Sodium: 416mg; Calcium: 203mg; Carbohydrates: 7g; Protein: 42g

1. Preheat the broiler.
2. Place the red pepper in a small baking dish and broil until blackened on all sides, turning as necessary. Transfer the pepper to a small bowl, and wrap the bowl tightly with plastic wrap. Let the pepper steam for 10 minutes. Peel off the skin, halve, and seed it, and add the pepper to a blender.
3. Add the sun-dried tomatoes, garlic, olive oil, lemon juice, cumin, coriander, caraway seeds, and salt. Purée until smooth.
4. Reduce the oven temperature to 400°F.
5. In a 9-by-9-inch baking dish, place the fillets in a single layer. Coat each piece generously with the harissa.
6. Bake for about 25 minutes until the fish is just cooked through. Serve.

SIMPLIFY IT: Harissa is a lovely ingredient for dips, sauces, and many other culinary applications. Double the recipe, and refrigerate this pretty condiment in a sealed container for up to 2 weeks.

PANFRIED TILAPIA
WITH COMPOUND BUTTER

Serves 4 | Prep time: 15 minutes, plus 2 hours chilling time | Cook time: 12 minutes

The beauty of compound butter is that it melts slowly when placed on a warm piece of fish, chicken, or meat, creating a delightful pool of flavor. Grass-fed butter contains vitamin K$_2$ (menaquinone), which is found in animal foods and helps keep calcium out of the arteries. Butter is also loaded with the anti-inflammatory fatty acid, butyrate (or butyric acid).

BRAIN BOOSTER
GLUTEN-FREE
IMMUNE BOOSTER
NUT-FREE
PALEO-FRIENDLY

For the compound butter
½ cup (1 stick) grass-fed butter
Zest of 1 orange
Juice of 1 orange
2 tablespoons chopped fresh thyme leaves
1 pinch Himalayan salt or table salt

For the fish
4 (6-ounce) tilapia fillets
Himalayan salt or table salt, for seasoning
Freshly ground black pepper, for seasoning
1 tablespoon extra-virgin olive oil

To make the compound butter

1. In a medium bowl, beat together the butter, orange zest and juice, thyme, and salt with an electric hand mixer until fluffy and blended.

2. Place a piece of plastic wrap on a clean work surface, and spoon the butter mixture into the center of the plastic wrap.

3. Fold one side of the plastic wrap over the butter, and roll the butter to form a log shape. Twist the ends of the plastic wrap to form a tight roll.

4. Refrigerate the butter for about 2 hours, until very firm.

To make the fish

1. Pat the fish dry with paper towels, and lightly season with salt and pepper.

2. In a large skillet over medium-high heat, heat the olive oil.

3. Add the fish. Pan-sear for about 12 minutes, turning once halfway through, until both sides are golden and the fish is cooked through. Transfer the fish to plates.

4. Slice the compound butter into ¾-inch disks. Top each fillet with butter and serve.

SIMPLIFY IT: Compound butters can be kept refrigerated for up to 1 week and frozen for up to 1 month, so whip up this flavorful topping ahead. Thaw the butter log a little, if frozen, before slicing it into disks.

Per Serving: **Calories:** 377; **Saturated Fat:** 14g; **Cholesterol:** 144mg; **Sodium:** 341mg; **Calcium:** 67mg; **Carbohydrates:** 1g; **Protein:** 32g

SPICE-RUBBED FLOUNDER WITH CITRUS SALSA

Serves 4 | Prep time: 20 minutes | Cook time: 10 minutes

Wild-caught flounder is very high in protein, like most fish, and contains all the essential amino acids as well as calcium. Flounder is rich in lysine, a crucial component for cell growth, calcium absorption, and muscle recovery. This fish is also a good source of nonessential amino acids linked to learning, memory, and cognitive function.

BRAIN BOOSTER
DAIRY-FREE
GLUTEN-FREE
IMMUNE BOOSTER
NUT-FREE
PALEO-FRIENDLY

For the citrus salsa

1 ruby red grapefruit, peeled, segmented, and coarsely chopped

1 orange, peeled, segmented, and coarsely chopped

2 celery stalks, chopped

1 scallion, white and green parts, chopped

2 tablespoons chopped fresh cilantro leaves

1 teaspoon grated lemon zest

Pinch Himalayan salt or table salt

For the fish

1 teaspoon ground cumin

½ teaspoon ground coriander

¼ teaspoon paprika

Pinch cayenne pepper

4 (6-ounce) flounder fillets, patted dry

2 tablespoons extra-virgin olive oil

To make the citrus salsa

1. In a small bowl, gently stir together the grapefruit, orange, celery, scallion, cilantro, and lemon zest.
2. Season the salsa with salt, and set it aside.

To make the fish

1. Preheat the oven to 425°F.
2. In a small bowl, stir together the cumin, coriander, paprika, and cayenne.
3. Rub both sides of the fillets with the spice mixture, and arrange them on a rimmed baking sheet.
4. Drizzle the fish with olive oil.
5. Bake the fish for about 10 minutes, until it is lightly golden and just cooked through.
6. Serve with the salsa.

Per Serving: Calories: 318; Saturated Fat: 3g; Cholesterol: 116mg; Sodium: 246mg; Calcium: 84mg; Carbohydrates: 12g; Protein: 42g

COCONUT MILK-BAKED CATFISH

Serves 4 | Prep time: 20 minutes | Cook time: 30 minutes

It is a very good thing that the sunny flavorful sauce this fish bakes in is thick because you will want to scrape up every last bit with your spoon. Saffron is mentioned in ancient writings as a treatment for many conditions, including stomach ailments and insomnia. This rare spice is high in vitamins B₆ and C, magnesium, and iron as well as more than 150 volatile compounds, including inflammation-fighting antioxidants and phytonutrients.

2 tablespoons warm water

Pinch saffron threads

1 pound catfish fillets

Himalayan salt or table salt, for seasoning

Freshly ground black pepper, for seasoning

1 tablespoon extra-virgin olive oil

1 sweet onion, chopped

2 teaspoons minced garlic

1 teaspoon grated fresh ginger

1 cup coconut milk

½ cup heavy (whipping) cream

2 tablespoons chopped fresh cilantro leaves

BRAIN BOOSTER
GLUTEN-FREE
IMMUNE BOOSTER

Per Serving: Calories: 494; Saturated Fat: 17g; Cholesterol: 112mg; Sodium: 392mg; Calcium: 83mg; Carbohydrates: 16g; Protein: 24g

1. Preheat the oven to 350°F.
2. Place the water in a small bowl, and sprinkle the saffron threads on top. Let it stand for 10 minutes.
3. Meanwhile, rub the catfish with salt and pepper, and place the fillets in a 9-by-9-inch baking dish.
4. Roast the fish for 10 minutes.
5. While the fish roasts, in a large skillet over medium-high heat, heat the olive oil.
6. Add the onion, garlic, and ginger. Sauté for about 3 minutes until softened.
7. Whisk in the coconut milk, heavy cream, and the saffron water. Bring the mixture to a boil, reduce the heat to low, and simmer the sauce for about 5 minutes until slightly thickened.
8. Pour the sauce over the fish, cover the baking dish, and bake the fish for 10 minutes more.
9. Serve topped with cilantro.

ROASTED TROUT WITH FENNEL

Serves 4 | Prep time: 20 minutes, plus 15 minutes pickling time | Cook time: 20 minutes

Fennel, a bulbous vegetable with dainty, frothy green fronds, tastes like licorice and combines very well with fish and seafood. It is a great source of fiber, vitamin C, potassium, magnesium, and copper. This vegetable is also rich in phytonutrients and antioxidants, such as quercitin and anethole, which reduce inflammation and the risk of degenerative diseases. The high vitamin C content fights free radicals that create the cellular damage that causes pain and joint deterioration.

½ cup apple cider vinegar

¼ cup water

1 tablespoon xylitol

1 teaspoon caraway seeds

1 teaspoon Himalayan salt or table salt

2 teaspoons minced garlic

1 fennel bulb, thinly sliced

1 carrot, shredded

4 (6-ounce) trout fillets

2 tablespoons extra-virgin olive oil

1 tablespoon freshly squeezed lemon juice

1 tablespoon chopped dill

BRAIN BOOSTER
DAIRY-FREE
GLUTEN-FREE
IMMUNE BOOSTER
NUT-FREE

1. Preheat the oven to 350°F.
2. In a small saucepan over medium heat, stir together the cider vinegar, water, xylitol, caraway seeds, and salt. Bring the mixture to a boil.
3. Transfer the liquid to a large bowl, and stir in the garlic. Set aside for 10 minutes.
4. Add the fennel and carrot to the liquid, and toss to coat. Let the mixture sit for about 15 minutes, until the fennel tastes pickled.
5. While the fennel pickles, arrange the trout in a 9-by-9-inch baking dish, and drizzle it with olive oil.
6. Roast the trout for about 15 minutes, until it flakes when lightly pressed.
7. Arrange the fennel mixture on 4 plates, and top each with a fillet.
8. Sprinkle each fillet with lemon juice and dill. Serve.

Per Serving: Calories: 433; Saturated Fat: 4g; Cholesterol: 126mg; Sodium: 527mg; Calcium: 154mg; Carbohydrates: 8g; Protein: 40g

BAKED SOLE
WITH PARSLEY PISTOU

Serves 4 | Prep time: 15 minutes | Cook time: 15 minutes

Pistou is an oil-based pesto-like sauce that typically features basil but can include all types of herbs, such as the parsley found in this recipe. Cashews provide bulk in the sauce as well as a healthy dose of monounsaturated fats, copper, magnesium, and zinc.

For the pistou

1 cup packed fresh parsley sprigs

¼ cup cashews

2 garlic cloves, lightly crushed

Zest of 1 lemon

Juice of 1 lemon

2 tablespoons extra-virgin olive oil

Pinch Himalayan salt or table salt

For the sole

4 (6-ounce) sole fillets

Himalayan salt or table salt, for seasoning

Freshly ground black pepper, for seasoning

1 tablespoon extra-virgin olive oil

BRAIN BOOSTER
DAIRY-FREE
GLUTEN-FREE
IMMUNE BOOSTER
PALEO-FRIENDLY

To make the pistou

1. In a blender, combine the parsley, cashews, garlic, lemon zest and juice, and olive oil. Pulse until a thick paste forms.
2. Season the pistou with salt, transfer to a bowl, and set aside.

To make the sole

1. Preheat the oven to 400°F.
2. Lightly season the fish with salt and pepper.
3. In a large ovenproof skillet over medium-high heat, heat the olive oil.
4. Add the fillets and pan-sear for 2 minutes on each side. Transfer the skillet to the oven.
5. Bake the fish for about 10 minutes, until just cooked through.
6. Serve the sole topped with a spoonful of pistou.

Per Serving: Calories: 340; Saturated Fat: 3g; Cholesterol: 116mg; Sodium: 267mg; Calcium: 43mg; Carbohydrates: 4g; Protein: 42g

TOMATO-BAKED BASS

Serves 4 | Prep time: 20 minutes | Cook time: 35 minutes

Baking fish right in a rich sauce is an ideal method of infusing the flesh with flavor and keeping it moist. Tomatoes and peppers are a pleasing pairing, especially when you add earthy kale and a generous sprinkling of fresh basil. These colorful veggies are high in all the inflammation-fighting antioxidants and phytonutrients needed for good health. The healthy fats from the olive oil round out the dish beautifully.

4 (6-ounce) bass fillets

3 tablespoons extra-virgin olive oil, plus more for the baking dish

1 sweet onion, thinly sliced

2 teaspoons minced garlic

5 tomatoes, diced

1 zucchini, diced

1 red bell pepper, diced

1 cup chopped kale

2 tablespoons chopped fresh basil leaves

BRAIN BOOSTER
DAIRY-FREE
GLUTEN-FREE
IMMUNE BOOSTER
NUT-FREE
PALEO-FRIENDLY

1. Preheat the oven to 400°F.
2. Lightly oil a 9-by-13-inch baking dish, and arrange the fish in a single layer. Set aside.
3. In a large skillet over medium-high heat, heat the olive oil.
4. Add the onion and garlic. Sauté for about 5 minutes, until lightly caramelized.
5. Stir in the tomatoes, zucchini, red bell pepper, and kale. Sauté for about 10 minutes more. Remove the skillet from heat, and spoon the tomato mixture over the fish.
6. Bake for 15 to 20 minutes, until the fish flakes easily.
7. Serve the fish garnished with the basil.

Per Serving: Calories: 405; Saturated Fat: 4g; Cholesterol: 148mg; Sodium: 175mg; Calcium: 232mg; Carbohydrates: 15g; Protein: 44g

ROASTED BELL PEPPER TROUT

Serves 4 | Prep time: 20 minutes | Cook time: 25 minutes

Trout is a small freshwater fish that features sweet flaky flesh and is usually available in most grocery stores. The fish is extremely rich in protein and omega-3 fatty acids and so is appropriate for a fibromyalgia diet. Protein can help you feel satiated longer and provide energy by fueling your muscles. Protein also reduces pain by repairing damage in the muscles' cells. Omega-3 fatty acids are anti-inflammatory and reduce the risk of depression.

BRAIN BOOSTER
DAIRY-FREE
GLUTEN-FREE
IMMUNE BOOSTER
NUT-FREE
PALEO-FRIENDLY

For the relish

1 red bell pepper, halved and seeded

1 orange bell pepper, halved and seeded

1 yellow bell pepper, halved and seeded

1 zucchini, halved lengthwise

3 tablespoons extra-virgin olive oil

Himalayan salt or table salt, for seasoning

Freshly ground black pepper, for seasoning

1 scallion, white and green parts, chopped

1 tablespoon apple cider vinegar

1 teaspoon chopped fresh basil leaves

For the fish

4 (6-ounce) trout fillets

Himalayan salt or table salt, for seasoning

Freshly ground black pepper, for seasoning

1 tablespoon extra-virgin olive oil

To make the relish

1. Preheat the broiler.
2. In a large bowl, toss the red, orange, and yellow bell peppers and zucchini with the olive oil. Season with salt and pepper, and arrange the vegetables on a rimmed baking sheet.
3. Broil for about 10 minutes, until the vegetables are lightly charred and tender, turning once about halfway through.
4. Remove the vegetables from the oven. Place the pepper halves in a small stainless steel bowl. Cover the bowl tightly with plastic wrap, and set aside for 10 minutes to steam. Peel off the skins.
5. Chop the peppers and zucchini, and transfer them to a small bowl.
6. Stir in the scallion, cider vinegar, and basil to mix. Set aside.

To make the fish

1. Pat the fish dry with paper towels, and season it with salt and pepper.
2. Place the fish in a baking dish, and drizzle with the olive oil.
3. Roast the fish for about 15 minutes, until it is just cooked through.
4. Serve the fish with the roasted pepper relish.

Per Serving: Calories: 383; Saturated Fat: 3g; Cholesterol: 0mg; Sodium: 125mg; Calcium: 23mg; Carbohydrates: 9g; Protein: 36g

SOLE WITH
GINGER-WASABI GLAZE

Serves 4 | Prep time: 15 minutes | Cook time: 20 minutes

It helps to be a fan of spicy food if you plan to make this flavorful dish, because wasabi definitely has a kick to it. Wasabi contains powerful antioxidant isothiocyanate compounds that reduce inflammation in the joints, ligaments, and muscles, crucial for fibromyalgia sufferers. Wasabi is also high in vitamins A and C, magnesium, iron, and calcium.

4 (6-ounce) sole fillets

2 tablespoons coconut aminos, divided

2 tablespoons coconut oil

2 tablespoons freshly squeezed orange juice

1 tablespoon grated orange zest

1 tablespoon wasabi paste

2 teaspoons grated fresh ginger

1 teaspoon xylitol

1 tablespoon chopped fresh cilantro

BRAIN BOOSTER
DAIRY-FREE
GLUTEN-FREE
IMMUNE BOOSTER

1. Preheat the oven to 400°F.
2. In a baking dish, arrange the fish and drizzle with 1 tablespoon coconut aminos. Set aside.
3. In a small bowl, stir together the remaining tablespoon coconut aminos, the coconut oil, orange juice and zest, wasabi paste, ginger, and xylitol until well blended. Coat the fish with the ginger-wasabi paste.
4. Bake the fish for about 20 minutes, until it is cooked through and the glaze is bubbly.
5. Serve topped with the cilantro.

COOKING TIP: The wasabi used in this recipe is the pale green Japanese variety sold as a paste or powder. If you can't find authentic wasabi, substitute horseradish, which is a member of the same family and is called wasabi-daikon.

Per Serving: Calories: 239; Saturated Fat: 3g; Cholesterol: 0mg; Sodium: 9mg; Calcium: 0mg; Carbohydrates: 4g; Protein: 31g

BAKED TILAPIA WITH
BLUEBERRY-AVOCADO SALSA

Serves 4 | Prep time: 20 minutes | Cook time: 15 minutes

Fresh salsa and fish are an absolutely charming combination. Fish is a magnificent source of cell-repairing protein, and the blueberries, walnuts, and avocado in the salsa are recommended for a diet designed to reduce fibromyalgia symptoms. These ingredients fight inflammation, increase sleep quality, and clear mental fog.

For the salsa

2 cups fresh blueberries
1 avocado, peeled, pitted, and diced
½ English cucumber, diced
½ cup chopped walnuts
½ cup chopped red onion
¼ cup chopped fresh cilantro leaves
Zest of 1 lime
Juice of 1 lime

For the fish

4 (6-ounce) tilapia fillets
Himalayan salt or table salt, for seasoning
Freshly ground black pepper, for seasoning
1 tablespoon extra-virgin olive oil

BRAIN BOOSTER
DAIRY-FREE
GLUTEN-FREE
IMMUNE BOOSTER
PALEO-FRIENDLY

To make the salsa

In a small bowl, stir together the blueberries, avocado, cucumber, walnuts, red onion, cilantro, and lime zest and juice. Set aside.

To make the fish

1. Preheat the oven to 350°F.
2. Pat the fish dry with paper towels, and season with salt and pepper. Place the fish in a 9-by-9-inch baking dish, and drizzle with the olive oil.
3. Bake the fish for about 15 minutes, until it is just cooked through.
4. Serve with the blueberry-avocado salsa.

Per Serving: Calories: 502; Saturated Fat: 5g; Cholesterol: 100mg; Sodium: 624mg; Calcium: 73mg; Carbohydrates: 19g; Protein: 50g

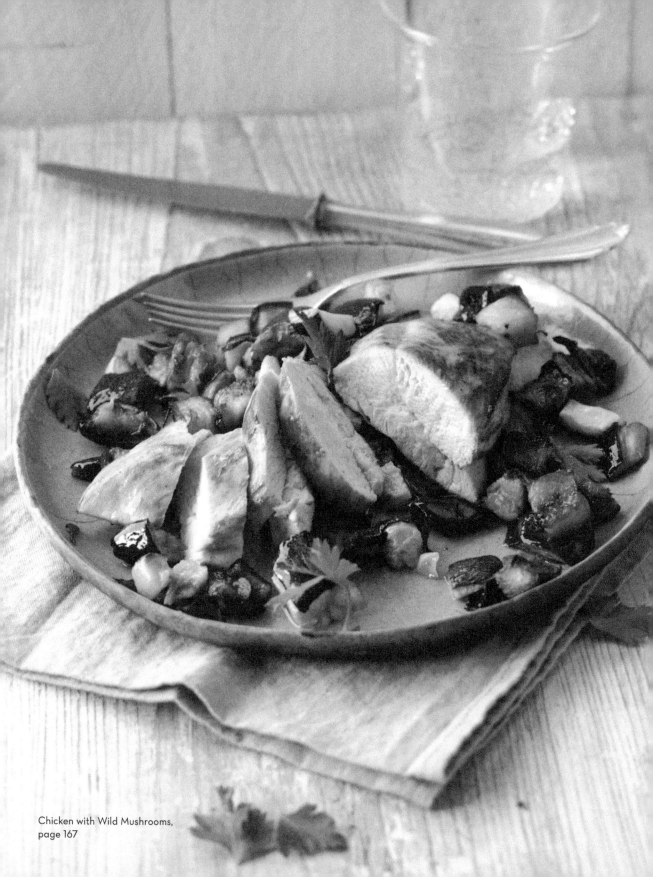

Chicken with Wild Mushrooms,
page 167

10

meat & poultry entrées

CREAMY SAFFRON
CHICKEN 166

CHICKEN WITH WILD
MUSHROOMS 167

EASY CHICKEN
PAD THAI 168

CHICKEN BREASTS WITH
RASPBERRY SAUCE 170

CHICKEN CACCIATORE 172

COCONUT MILK-BRAISED
CHICKEN 173

TURKEY, LEEK, AND
PUMPKIN CASSEROLE 174

TURKEY STROGANOFF 175

TURKEY SHEPHERD'S
PIE 176

TURKEY CHILI 178

PORK TENDERLOIN WITH
CARAMELIZED ONIONS 179

ROASTED VENISON
LEG 180

MUSTARD-CRUSTED
VENISON 181

LAMB-VEGETABLE
STEW 182

ACORN SQUASH
LAMB GRATIN 184

TRADITIONAL HERBED
MEATLOAF 186

ZUCCHINI PASTA WITH
BEEF AND EGGPLANT
SAUCE 187

BEEF CHOW MEIN 188

BEEF POT ROAST
WITH VEGETABLES 190

ITALIAN-STYLE
MEATBALLS 191

CREAMY SAFFRON CHICKEN

Serves 4 | Prep time: 10 minutes, plus 1 hour marinating time and 15 minutes resting time
Cook time: 20 minutes

Yogurt is very high in calcium, a mineral often deficient in those with fibromyalgia. Calcium can help alleviate muscle soreness and spasms, general aches and pains, and insomnia. Balance your calcium intake with magnesium, found in foods such as pumpkin seeds, dark chocolate, and coriander. Magnesium and calcium work together, allowing the muscles to contract and relax.

1 cup plain, full-fat yogurt
1 teaspoon minced garlic
¼ teaspoon Himalayan salt or table salt
Pinch saffron threads
4 (6-ounce) boneless skinless chicken breasts, halved lengthwise
Olive oil spray, for coating the baking sheet

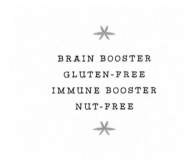

BRAIN BOOSTER
GLUTEN-FREE
IMMUNE BOOSTER
NUT-FREE

Per Serving: Calories: 206; Saturated Fat: 1g; Cholesterol: 94mg; Sodium: 232mg; Calcium: 121mg; Carbohydrates: 4g; Protein: 34g

1. In a large bowl, whisk the yogurt, garlic, salt, and saffron until well blended.
2. Add the chicken breasts, turning to coat each piece thoroughly.
3. Refrigerator to marinate for 1 hour.
4. Preheat the broiler.
5. Spray a rimmed baking sheet with olive oil spray.
6. Remove the chicken breasts from the marinade, and place them on the prepared sheet. Let the tray stand at room temperature for 15 minutes.
7. Broil the chicken for about 10 minutes, turn, and continue broiling for 10 minutes more, until golden and cooked through. Serve.

A CLOSER LOOK: Saffron adds glorious flavor and a lovely yellow color to the dish. Saffron threads are the stigmas from crocus flowers—about 5,000 threads per ounce! Real saffron has a lighter tip than the rest of the thread rather than a uniform color, which indicates dyed stigmas from other flowers.

CHICKEN WITH WILD MUSHROOMS

Serves 4 | Prep time: 20 minutes | Cook time: 35 minutes

Chicken breast is a fantastic source of protein, which repairs damaged muscle cells, thus relieving pain while fueling those same muscles to provide needed energy. Portobello mushrooms add vitamin D to this dish, whose deficiency has been linked to health problems such as musculoskeletal pain, high blood pressure, and osteoporosis.

4 (6-ounce) boneless skinless chicken breasts
Himalayan salt or table salt, for seasoning
Freshly ground black pepper, for seasoning
3 tablespoons extra-virgin olive oil, divided
3 tablespoons grass-fed butter
2 large portobello mushrooms, diced
1 zucchini, diced
3 garlic cloves, sliced
Fresh flat leaf parsley sprigs, for garnish

BRAIN BOOSTER
GLUTEN-FREE
IMMUNE BOOSTER
NUT-FREE
PALEO-FRIENDLY

Per Serving: Calories: 506; Saturated Fat: 10g; Cholesterol: 174mg; Sodium: 241mg; Calcium: 42mg; Carbohydrates: 3g; Protein: 51g

1. Preheat the oven to 400°F.
2. Lightly season the chicken breasts with salt and pepper.
3. In a large ovenproof skillet over medium-high heat, heat 2 tablespoons olive oil.
4. Add the chicken breasts and brown for about 4 minutes per side. Transfer the skillet to the oven.
5. Roast the chicken for about 25 minutes until just cooked through.
6. When the chicken has been roasting for 10 minutes, heat the remaining tablespoon olive oil and melt the butter in a medium skillet over medium-high heat.
7. Add the mushrooms, zucchini, and garlic. Sauté for about 10 minutes, stirring frequently, until tender and lightly caramelized.
8. Serve the chicken breasts with a generous scoop of vegetables garnished with parsley.

EASY CHICKEN PAD THAI

Serves 4 | Prep time: 30 minutes | Cook time: 0 minutes

This dish is traditionally served with noodles made from rice or other grains but is equally delicious with these colorful veggie noodles. Loads of different vegetables, a generous portion of chicken, crunchy nuts, and a sauce created with healthy mono-unsaturated oils and antioxidant-packed ginger and garlic mean this is a meal that supports your fibromyalgia goals. Increase the red pepper flakes for more heat and greater amounts of pain-relieving capsaicin.

BRAIN BOOSTER
DAIRY-FREE
GLUTEN-FREE
IMMUNE BOOSTER

For the sauce

¼ cup freshly squeezed lime juice

2 tablespoons freshly squeezed orange juice

2 tablespoons sesame oil

2 tablespoons almond butter

1 tablespoon xylitol

2 teaspoons coconut aminos

1 teaspoon minced garlic

1 teaspoon grated fresh ginger

¼ teaspoon red pepper flakes

For the pad thai

1 zucchini, spiralized or julienned

1 yellow summer squash, spiralized or julienned

1 carrot, spiralized or julienned

1 red bell pepper, julienned

1 yellow bell pepper, julienned

2 cups bean sprouts

2 cups diced cooked chicken

2 tablespoons chopped cashews

1 scallion, white and green parts, thinly sliced on a bias

To make the sauce

In a small bowl, whisk the lime juice, orange juice, sesame oil, almond butter, xylitol, coconut aminos, garlic, ginger, and red pepper flakes until well blended. Set aside.

To make the pad thai

1. In a large bowl, toss together the zucchini, summer squash, carrot, red and yellow bell peppers, bean sprouts, and chicken.
2. Add the dressing, and toss until the vegetables and chicken are well coated.
3. Top with the cashews and scallion and serve.

Per Serving: **Calories:** 274; **Saturated Fat:** 2g; **Cholesterol:** 54mg; **Sodium:** 183mg; **Calcium:** 63mg; **Carbohydrates:** 18g; **Protein:** 30g

CHICKEN BREASTS WITH RASPBERRY SAUCE

Serves 4 | Prep time: 10 minutes | Cook time: 25 minutes

Fruit sauces, particularly berries, are perfect for meat and poultry dishes because the sweetness and acidity complement the protein's flavor and texture. Raspberries are considered a superfood due to their antioxidant content and anti-inflammatory phytonutrients, such as ellagic acid, quercetin, catechins, kaempferol, and salicylic acid.

BRAIN BOOSTER
DAIRY-FREE
GLUTEN-FREE
IMMUNE BOOSTER
NUT-FREE
PALEO-FRIENDLY

For the chicken

4 (6-ounce) boneless skinless chicken breasts
Himalayan salt or table salt, for seasoning
Freshly ground black pepper, for seasoning
2 tablespoons extra-virgin olive oil

For the sauce

2 tablespoons extra-virgin olive oil
2 shallots, minced
½ cup gluten-free, sodium-free chicken broth
2 tablespoons apple cider vinegar
1 cup fresh raspberries
¼ teaspoon ground nutmeg
1 teaspoon grated lemon zest

To make the chicken

1. Preheat the oven to 425°F.
2. Lightly season the chicken breasts with salt and pepper.
3. In a medium ovenproof skillet over medium-high heat, heat the olive oil.
4. Add the chicken and brown for about 5 minutes, turning once. Transfer the skillet to the oven.
5. Roast the chicken for about 20 minutes, until just cooked through. Remove from the oven, and let the chicken rest for 10 minutes.
6. Slice the chicken into medallions.

To make the sauce

1. While the chicken roasts, heat the olive oil in a small saucepan over medium-high heat.
2. Add the shallots. Sauté for about 3 minutes, until softened.
3. Stir in the chicken broth and cider vinegar. Bring the liquid to a boil, reduce the heat to low, and simmer for about 5 minutes, until the sauce is reduced by half.
4. Stir in the raspberries and nutmeg. Cook for about 5 minutes, until the berries break down. Remove the sauce from the heat, and stir in the lemon zest.
5. Serve the chicken topped with the raspberry sauce.

Per Serving: Calories: 304; Saturated Fat: 3g; Cholesterol: 91mg; Sodium: 132mg; Calcium: 23mg; Carbohydrates: 4g; Protein: 31g

CHICKEN CACCIATORE

Serves 4 | Prep time: 20 minutes | Cook time: 38 minutes

Cacciatore means "hunter" in Italian, and a hunter sauce in professional kitchens usually means a sauce prepared with mushrooms and tomatoes. There are no mushrooms in this variation, but the sun-dried tomatoes double up the appetizing, sweet tomato flavor. Sun-dried tomatoes are high in fiber, protein, and vitamin B₁₂. Sun-dried tomatoes can boost energy, support healthy digestion, and help reduce muscle pain.

3 tablespoons extra-virgin olive oil

4 (5-ounce) boneless skinless chicken breasts, halved horizontally

Himalayan salt or table salt, for seasoning

Freshly ground black pepper, for seasoning

1 sweet onion, chopped

1 tablespoon minced garlic

2 (28-ounce) cans sodium-free diced tomatoes

1 cup sun-dried tomatoes, chopped

2 tablespoons chopped fresh basil leaves

1 tablespoon chopped fresh oregano leaves

¼ teaspoon red pepper flakes

2 tablespoons chopped fresh parsley leaves

BRAIN BOOSTER
DAIRY-FREE
GLUTEN-FREE
IMMUNE BOOSTER
NUT-FREE
PALEO-FRIENDLY

1. In a large skillet over medium-high heat, heat the olive oil.
2. Season the chicken lightly with salt and pepper. Add it to the skillet and sauté for about 5 minutes per side. Transfer the chicken to a plate and set aside.
3. Return the skillet to the heat. Add the onion and garlic. Sauté for about 3 minutes until softened.
4. Stir in the tomatoes, sun-dried tomatoes, basil, oregano, and red pepper flakes. Bring the sauce to a boil, and return the chicken to the skillet. Reduce the heat to low, and simmer for about 25 minutes, until the chicken is cooked through.
5. Serve topped with the parsley.

A CLOSER LOOK: Parsley is a spectacular source of chlorophyll, and vitamins A, C, and K, as well as beta-carotene, iron, calcium, potassium, and zinc. This herb supports the immune system, purifies the blood, and cuts the risk of diabetes, atherosclerosis, and stroke.

Per Serving: Calories: 373; Saturated Fat: 3g; Cholesterol: 91mg; Sodium: 436mg; Calcium: 92mg; Carbohydrates: 27g; Protein: 36g

COCONUT MILK-BRAISED CHICKEN

Serves 4 | Prep time: 10 minutes | Cook time: 40 minutes

Braising is a traditional culinary technique that uses moist and dry heat, and is usually completed in a sealed vessel in the oven. The lightly spiced coconut milk in this recipe infuses the chicken with moisture and flavor while adding naturally occurring electrolytes that support muscle health, and lauric acid that boosts the immune system. Cumin, cinnamon, and cloves are also delicious additions to the spiced coconut milk.

1 cup coconut milk

½ cup heavy (whipping) cream

Zest of 1 lime

Juice of 1 lime

2 tablespoons grated fresh ginger

1 tablespoon xylitol

½ teaspoon ground turmeric

½ teaspoon ground cardamom

1 tablespoon extra-virgin olive oil

1 pound chicken thighs

2 tablespoons chopped fresh cilantro leaves

Freshly ground black pepper, for seasoning

BRAIN BOOSTER
GLUTEN-FREE
IMMUNE BOOSTER

1. In a medium bowl, whisk the coconut milk, heavy cream, lime zest and juice, ginger, xylitol, turmeric, and cardamom until well blended. Set aside.

2. In a large skillet over medium-high heat, heat the olive oil.

3. Add the chicken, and pan-sear for about 20 minutes, until golden, turning once about halfway through.

4. Pour in the spiced coconut milk, and bring the liquid to a boil. Reduce the heat to low, cover, and simmer the chicken for about 20 minutes, until it is tender and cooked through.

5. Serve garnished with cilantro and seasoned with pepper.

Per Serving: Calories: 446; Saturated Fat: 19g; Cholesterol: 121mg; Sodium: 113mg; Calcium: 43mg; Carbohydrates: 6g; Protein: 35g

TURKEY, LEEK, AND PUMPKIN CASSEROLE

Serves 4 | Prep time: 25 minutes | Cook time: 40 minutes

Casseroles are great time-saving creations for when you want to make something ahead or throw a satisfying meal together quickly. This casserole is seasoned with pink Himalayan salt, which can prevent muscle cramps, lower blood pressure, and increase metabolism.

3 tablespoons extra-virgin olive oil,
    plus extra for oiling the casserole dish
1 pound ground turkey
2 leeks, white part only, roots trimmed and
    tough outer leaves removed, well cleaned,
    and thinly sliced crosswise
2 teaspoons minced garlic
1 pound chopped pumpkin
2 cups cauliflower florets
1 tablespoon chopped fresh thyme leaves
Himalayan salt or table salt, for seasoning
Freshly ground black pepper, for seasoning

BRAIN BOOSTER
DAIRY-FREE
GLUTEN-FREE
IMMUNE BOOSTER
NUT-FREE
PALEO-FRIENDLY

Per Serving: Calories: 393; Saturated Fat: 4g;
Cholesterol: 115mg; Sodium: 210mg; Calcium: 114mg;
Carbohydrates: 19g; Protein: 34g

1. Preheat the oven to 350°F.
2. Lightly oil a large casserole dish with olive oil.
3. In a large skillet over medium-high heat, heat the olive oil.
4. Add the turkey. Sauté for about 6 minutes, breaking it up with the back of a spoon, until cooked through.
5. Add the leeks and garlic. Sauté for about 5 minutes, until softened.
6. Stir in the pumpkin and cauliflower, and cook for 3 minutes.
7. Remove the skillet from the heat, stir in the thyme, and season the mixture with salt and pepper.
8. Transfer the mixture to the prepared dish, and bake for about 25 minutes, until the vegetables are tender.

SIMPLIFY IT: Assemble the casserole through step 8 into the dish. Cover and refrigerator the casserole for up to 1 day if you want a quick meal with no cleanup. Bake the casserole, and add 15 minutes to the cooking time.

TURKEY STROGANOFF

Serves 4 | Prep time: 15 minutes | Cook time: 30 minutes

Stroganoff is comfort food—rich, creamy, and studded with lots of mushrooms. This dish is often made with beef, but turkey is a lovely alternative. Dijon mustard adds a distinctive flavor to the sauce and a plethora of nutrients. Mustard is part of the cruciferous vegetable family. It shouldn't be surprising, then, that it is high in phytonutrients, selenium, and magnesium. Magnesium is linked to pain relief, selenium can improve sleep quality, and mustard can help reduce body-wide inflammation.

3 tablespoons extra-virgin olive oil

1 pound turkey breast, cut into 1-inch chunks

1 sweet onion, chopped

2 teaspoons minced garlic

8 ounces button mushrooms, sliced

2 cups gluten-free, sodium-free chicken broth

2 tablespoons arrowroot powder

1 tablespoon Dijon mustard

1 teaspoon chopped fresh thyme leaves

½ cup heavy (whipping) cream

Himalayan salt or table salt, for seasoning

Freshly ground black pepper, for seasoning

2 tablespoons chopped fresh parsley leaves

BRAIN BOOSTER
GLUTEN-FREE
IMMUNE BOOSTER
NUT-FREE

1. In a large skillet over medium-high heat, heat the olive oil.
2. Add the turkey and sauté for about 10 minutes, until cooked through and lightly browned. Using a slotted spoon, transfer the turkey to a plate.
3. Return the skillet to the heat, and add the onion and garlic. Sauté for 3 minutes.
4. Add the mushrooms. Sauté for 5 minutes.
5. Whisk in the chicken broth, arrowroot powder, mustard, and thyme. Cook for about 10 minutes, whisking until the sauce thickens.
6. Return the turkey to the skillet, and add the heavy cream. Season with salt and pepper.
7. Serve sprinkled with the parsley.

Per Serving: Calories: 309; Saturated Fat: 5g; Cholesterol: 69mg; Sodium: 932mg; Calcium: 43mg; Carbohydrates: 11g; Protein: 22g

TURKEY SHEPHERD'S PIE

Serves 4 | Prep time: 20 minutes | Cook time: 1 hour

Turkey is known for its tryptophan content, and many people have experienced its effects after a large roast turkey dinner when they end up on the couch, snoring. Tryptophan is a precursor to an essential brain chemical, serotonin. Including foods in your diet that are high in tryptophan is a good strategy for managing your symptoms.

BRAIN BOOSTER
GLUTEN-FREE
IMMUNE BOOSTER
NUT-FREE

3 sweet potatoes, peeled and cut
    into 2-inch chunks
¼ cup heavy (whipping) cream
2 tablespoons grass-fed butter
Himalayan salt or table salt, for seasoning
Freshly ground black pepper, for seasoning
1 tablespoon extra-virgin olive oil
1 pound ground turkey
2 celery stalks, chopped
½ sweet onion, chopped
2 teaspoons minced garlic
2 carrots, cut into disks
2 cups small cauliflower florets
1 teaspoon chopped fresh thyme leaves

1. In a large saucepan over medium-high heat, combine the sweet potatoes and enough cold water to cover by about 2 inches. Bring to a boil, reduce the heat to low, and simmer for about 20 minutes, until the potatoes are tender. Drain the sweet potatoes and return them to the pot.
2. Add the heavy cream and butter. Mash until very fluffy. Season with salt and pepper and set aside.
3. Preheat the oven to 350°F.
4. In a large skillet over medium-high heat, heat the olive oil.
5. Add the turkey. Cook for about 10 minutes, breaking it up with the back of a spoon, until cooked through.
6. Add the celery, onion, and garlic. Sauté for about 3 minutes, until softened.
7. Add the carrots and cauliflower. Sauté for about 10 minutes.
8. Stir in the thyme, and spoon the turkey mixture into a 9-by-13-inch baking dish.
9. Spread the mashed sweet potatoes evenly over the top.
10. Bake the casserole for about 20 minutes, until bubbling and lightly browned. Serve.

Per Serving: Calories: 514; Saturated Fat: 6g; Cholesterol: 134mg; Sodium: 202mg; Calcium: 97mg; Carbohydrates: 45g; Protein: 36g

TURKEY CHILI

Serves 5 | Prep time: 20 minutes | Cook time: 40 minutes

Chili is the focus of festivals and secret recipe contests because the right combination of ingredients creates culinary magic. The addition of sweet squash and mushrooms ensures more than enough bulk to soak up the fiery spices. Chili powder is incredibly high in capsaicin, so chili can positively affect the pain associated with fibromyalgia.

3 tablespoons extra-virgin olive oil

2 pounds ground turkey

2 sweet onions, chopped

2 cups halved button mushrooms

4 teaspoons minced garlic

1 green bell pepper, diced

1 red bell pepper, diced

2 cups diced butternut squash

4 tablespoons chili powder

½ teaspoon ground cumin

Pinch cayenne pepper

2 (28-ounce) cans sodium-free diced tomatoes

Himalayan salt or table salt, for seasoning

Freshly ground black pepper, for seasoning

¼ cup plain, full-fat yogurt

1 scallion, white and green parts, thinly sliced on a bias

BRAIN BOOSTER
GLUTEN-FREE
IMMUNE BOOSTER
NUT-FREE

1. In a large saucepan over medium-high heat, heat the olive oil.
2. Add the turkey. Sauté for about 10 minutes, breaking it up with the back of a spoon, until cooked through.
3. Add the onions, mushrooms, and garlic. Sauté for 5 minutes.
4. Add the green and red bell peppers, butternut squash, chili powder, cumin, and cayenne. Sauté for about 4 minutes, stirring to coat everything with the spices.
5. Add the tomatoes and bring the mixture to a boil. Reduce the heat to low, and simmer for about 20 minutes, until the vegetables are tender.
6. Season the chili with salt and pepper. Serve topped with the yogurt and scallion.

COOKING TIP: Chili can be made with any type of ground meat instead of the turkey in this spicy dish. If you want to duplicate real Texas-style chili, use diced beef cubes and braise them for several hours in the spicy sauce until very tender.

Per Serving: Calories: 592; Saturated Fat: 6g; Cholesterol: 186mg; Sodium: 287mg; Calcium: 172mg; Carbohydrates: 29g; Protein: 57g

PORK TENDERLOIN
WITH CARAMELIZED ONIONS

Serves 4 | Prep time: 10 minutes | Cook time: 20 minutes

Pork is a juicy, budget-friendly protein choice that is easy to cook and pairs well with other ingredients like these golden sweet onions. Pork is also a good source of the amino acid L-carnitine, crucial for supporting tissue strength and promoting growth and effective healing in muscles.

3 tablespoons extra-virgin olive oil, divided

1 tablespoon grass-fed butter

2 sweet onions, halved lengthwise
   and thinly sliced

1 teaspoon minced garlic

1 teaspoon chopped fresh thyme leaves

2 (12-ounce) pork tenderloins, trimmed

Himalayan salt or table salt, for seasoning

Freshly ground black pepper, for seasoning

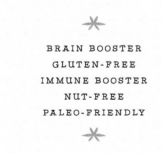

BRAIN BOOSTER
GLUTEN-FREE
IMMUNE BOOSTER
NUT-FREE
PALEO-FRIENDLY

Per Serving: Calories: 382; Saturated Fat: 5g; Cholesterol: 132mg; Sodium: 120mg; Calcium: 32mg; Carbohydrates: 5g; Protein: 45g

1. Preheat the oven to 400°F.
2. In a large skillet over medium heat, heat 2 tablespoons olive oil and melt the butter.
3. Add the onions, garlic, and thyme. Sauté for about 20 minutes, stirring frequently, until the onions are golden and caramelized. Remove the skillet from the heat, cover, and set aside.
4. While the onions caramelize, season the pork all over with salt and pepper.
5. In a medium ovenproof skillet over medium-high heat, heat the remaining tablespoon olive oil.
6. Add the pork and brown for about 5 minutes, browning all sides. Transfer the skillet to the oven.
7. Roast the pork for about 15 minutes, until it is just cooked through.
8. Let the meat rest for 10 minutes before slicing and serving with the caramelized onions.

ROASTED VENISON LEG

Serves 4 | Prep time: 10 minutes, plus 30 minutes resting time | Cook time: 50 minutes

The flavorful paste used in this recipe, plus cooking by searing, ensures the venison retains incredible moisture and appetizing color. Venison is high in protein, vitamins B$_{12}$ and B$_6$, and iron, which is essential for brain health and healthy muscles.

½ cup fresh mint leaves

¼ cup fresh cilantro leaves

5 garlic cloves

1 teaspoon cumin seeds

Zest of 1 lime

Juice of 1 lime

3 tablespoons extra-virgin olive oil

2 pounds boneless venison leg

1 cup gluten-free, sodium-free chicken broth

¼ cup balsamic vinegar

1 tablespoon xylitol

BRAIN BOOSTER
DAIRY-FREE
GLUTEN-FREE
IMMUNE BOOSTER
NUT-FREE

Per Serving: Calories: 274; Saturated Fat: 3g; Cholesterol: 0mg; Sodium: 120mg; Calcium: 43mg; Carbohydrates: 3g; Protein: 26g

1. Preheat the oven to 375°F.
2. In a blender, combine the mint, cilantro, garlic, cumin seeds, lime zest and juice, and olive oil. Blend until a paste forms.
3. Slather the paste all over the venison leg, and let the meat sit for 30 minutes at room temperature.
4. Heat a large ovenproof skillet over medium-high heat. Add the venison and pan-sear for about 7 minutes, browning all sides. Transfer the leg to a roasting pan.
5. Roast the venison for about 35 minutes for medium-rare, or to your desired doneness. Remove the meat from the roasting pan, and place it on a plate to rest.
6. Place the roasting pan over medium heat, and stir in the chicken broth, balsamic vinegar, and xylitol. Bring the liquid to a boil, reduce the heat to low, and simmer for about 6 minutes until the sauce reduces by half.
7. Slice the venison, and serve drizzled with the sauce.

MUSTARD-CRUSTED VENISON

Serves 4 | Prep time: 15 minutes | Cook time: 12 minutes

Rosemary's distinctive flavor means it pairs perfectly with strong-tasting meats. In this recipe, rosemary is complemented by thyme and tangy Dijon mustard to create a classic crust. Rosemary contains many anti-inflammatory and anti-oxidant compounds, including rosmarinic acid, a potent free-radical fighter. When the herb is heated, as with this juicy piece of venison, the action of these important compounds increases.

2 cups finely chopped pistachios

½ cup finely chopped cashews

2 teaspoons chopped fresh rosemary leaves

1 teaspoon chopped fresh thyme leaves

⅛ teaspoon Himalayan salt or table salt

⅛ teaspoon freshly ground black pepper

½ cup grainy Dijon mustard

24 ounces venison tenderloin,
   cut into 8 medallions

Olive oil spray, for coating the venison

BRAIN BOOSTER
DAIRY-FREE
GLUTEN-FREE
IMMUNE BOOSTER
PALEO-FRIENDLY

1. Preheat the oven to 400°F.
2. In a medium bowl, stir together the pistachios, cashews, rosemary, thyme, salt, and pepper.
3. Brush the venison medallions on both sides with mustard, and dredge the meat in the nut mixture. Arrange the medallions on a rimmed baking sheet, and lightly spray both sides of each piece with olive oil spray.
4. Roast the meat for about 12 minutes for medium-rare, turning once, until the crust is golden and the meat is cooked to your desired doneness.
5. Let the meat rest for 10 minutes, and serve 2 medallions per person.

Per Serving (2 medallions): **Calories:** 535; **Saturated Fat:** 5g; **Cholesterol:** 150mg; **Sodium:** 615mg; **Calcium:** 92mg; **Carbohydrates:** 15g; **Protein:** 60g

LAMB-VEGETABLE STEW

Serves 4 | Prep time: 15 minutes | Cook time: 1 hour, 45 minutes

Lamb is a popular protein choice, especially in countries that do not have a thriving beef industry. This healthy meat is rich in protein, omega-3 fatty acids, and conjugated linoleic acid (CLA), and has more than 100 percent of the RDA of vitamin B_{12}. Eating lamb can reduce inflammation, increase metabolism and energy, and facilitate cell repair in muscles. Lamb has also been linked to better blood sugar regulation.

BRAIN BOOSTER
DAIRY-FREE
GLUTEN-FREE
IMMUNE BOOSTER
NUT-FREE
PALEO-FRIENDLY

3 tablespoons extra-virgin olive oil

1 pound lamb shoulder, cut into ½-inch chunks

2 celery stalks, diced

1 sweet onion, chopped

2 teaspoons minced garlic

4 cups gluten-free, sodium-free beef broth

1 (28-ounce) can sodium-free diced tomatoes

2 carrots, diced

2 parsnips, diced

1 sweet potato, peeled and diced

1 cup shredded baby bok choy

1 tablespoon chopped fresh rosemary leaves

3 tablespoons water

2 tablespoons arrowroot powder

Himalayan salt or table salt, for seasoning

Freshly ground black pepper, for seasoning

1. In a large stockpot over medium-high heat, heat the olive oil.
2. Add the lamb and brown for about 10 minutes, browning all sides.
3. Add the celery, onion, and garlic. Sauté for 3 minutes.
4. Stir in the beef broth and tomatoes, and bring the liquid to a boil. Reduce the heat to low, and simmer for 1 hour.
5. Add the carrots, parsnips, and sweet potato. Simmer for about 15 minutes, until the vegetables are tender.
6. Stir in the bok choy and rosemary. Simmer for 10 minutes more.
7. In a small bowl, whisk the water and arrowroot powder until blended. Stir this mixture into the stew, and cook for about 4 minutes, stirring, until the broth thickens.
8. Season the stew with salt and pepper. Serve.

SIMPLIFY IT: This stew can be made in a slow cooker by stirring together all the ingredients, except the water and arrowroot powder. Cover and cook for 10 hours on low or for 5 hours on high heat. Add the arrowroot mixture to the stew after it is completely cooked, continuing to cook until heated through.

Per Serving: Calories: 464; Saturated Fat: 6g; Cholesterol: 102mg; Sodium: 161mg; Calcium: 112mg; Carbohydrates: 36g; Protein: 37g

ACORN SQUASH LAMB GRATIN

Serves 4 | Prep time: 25 minutes | Cook time: 45 minutes

When you remove this enchanting casserole from the oven, you might not want to disturb the golden melted cheese topping with your spoon or fork. Rich and decadent cream cheese and almonds combine here to crumbly perfection. Cream cheese has the fat required in a fibromyalgia diet along with protein, vitamins A and B$_{12}$, and calcium. These nutrients provide energy and help fight inflammation.

BRAIN BOOSTER
GLUTEN-FREE
IMMUNE BOOSTER

1 tablespoon extra-virgin olive oil, plus extra for oiling the casserole dish

1 pound ground lamb

2 celery stalks, chopped

½ sweet onion, chopped

2 teaspoons minced garlic

1 pound acorn squash, cut into 1-inch chunks

2 cups halved cherry tomatoes

2 tablespoons chopped fresh parsley leaves

Himalayan salt or table salt, for seasoning

Freshly ground black pepper, for seasoning

1 cup cream cheese, at room temperature

½ cup almond flour

1. Preheat the oven to 350°F.
2. Lightly oil a large casserole dish with olive oil.
3. In a large skillet over medium-high heat, heat the olive oil.
4. Add the lamb and sauté for about 6 minutes, breaking it up with the back of a spoon, until cooked through.
5. Add the celery, onion, and garlic. Sauté for about 4 minutes until softened.
6. Add the squash and sauté for 5 minutes more.
7. Remove the skillet from the heat, and stir in the tomatoes and parsley.
8. Season the mixture with salt and pepper, and transfer to the casserole dish.
9. In a small bowl, mix the cream cheese with the almond flour until the mixture resembles coarse crumbs. Sprinkle the cheese mixture over the casserole.
10. Bake for about 30 minutes, until the vegetables are very tender and the topping is bubbly and golden. Serve.

Per Serving: Calories: 583; Saturated Fat: 16g; Cholesterol: 166mg; Sodium: 274mg; Calcium: 154mg; Carbohydrates: 21g; Protein: 41g

TRADITIONAL HERBED MEATLOAF

Serves 4 | Prep time: 15 minutes | Cook time: 1 hour

Simple ground meats, herbs, an egg, and a splash of cream come together in a mouth-watering dish that might become a new family favorite. Meatloaf freezes beautifully, so make a double batch and set one aside in the freezer for a later meal. Onion may seem like a small part of the dish as with many other recipes, but this vegetable provides flavor and depth to the other ingredients. Onion is high in antioxidants such as quercetin that can fight cell-damaging inflammation and support general good health.

¾ pound ground beef

¾ pound ground pork

½ cup almond flour

1 egg

¼ cup heavy (whipping) cream

½ sweet onion, chopped

1 teaspoon minced garlic

1 tablespoon chopped fresh parsley leaves

1 teaspoon chopped fresh basil leaves

1 teaspoon chopped fresh oregano leaves

⅛ teaspoon Himalayan salt or table salt

⅛ teaspoon freshly ground black pepper

BRAIN BOOSTER
GLUTEN-FREE
IMMUNE BOOSTER

1. Preheat the oven to 350°F.
2. In a large bowl, mix the beef, pork, almond flour, egg, heavy cream, onion, garlic, parsley, basil, oregano, salt, and pepper until well combined. Press the meatloaf mixture into a 9-by-5-inch loaf pan.
3. Bake for about 1 hour, until cooked through.
4. Remove the meatloaf from the oven, and let it rest for 10 minutes.
5. Discard any excess grease, slice, and serve.

Per Serving: Calories: 409; Saturated Fat: 6g; Cholesterol: 189mg; Sodium: 125mg; Calcium: 43mg; Carbohydrates: 3g; Protein: 51g

ZUCCHINI PASTA WITH BEEF AND EGGPLANT SAUCE

Serves 4 | Prep time: 20 minutes | Cook time: 45 minutes

A delicious basic pasta sauce is a great addition to your culinary repertoire and can be used in casseroles or served over these nutritious zucchini noodles. Top this dish with a spoonful or two of full-fat cottage cheese for extra protein and calcium. Eggplant is a great source of vitamins B6 and C, fiber, manganese, copper, magnesium, and pantothenic acid. Several of these nutrients can help reduce pain and improve sleep.

3 tablespoons extra-virgin olive oil

1 pound ground beef

6 cups diced eggplant

½ sweet onion, chopped

1 tablespoon minced garlic

2 (28-ounce) cans sodium-free diced tomatoes

2 tablespoons chopped fresh basil leaves

1 tablespoon chopped fresh oregano leaves

½ teaspoon red pepper flakes

¼ teaspoon Himalayan salt or table salt

¼ teaspoon freshly ground black pepper

4 zucchini, spiralized or julienned

BRAIN BOOSTER
DAIRY-FREE
GLUTEN-FREE
IMMUNE BOOSTER
NUT-FREE
PALEO-FRIENDLY

1. In a large skillet over medium-high heat, heat the olive oil.
2. Add the ground beef and sauté for about 7 minutes, breaking it up with the back of a spoon, until cooked through.
3. Add the eggplant, onion, and garlic. Sauté for about 15 minutes, until the vegetables are tender.
4. Stir in the tomatoes, basil, oregano, red pepper flakes, salt, and pepper. Bring the sauce to a boil, reduce the heat to low, and simmer for about 20 minutes, until the flavors mellow and the eggplant chunks start to break apart.
5. Serve the sauce over the zucchini noodles.

SIMPLIFY IT: The zucchini noodles can be made several days ahead and kept refrigerated in a sealed container for up to 5 days. Pat the noodles dry with paper towels before using them.

Per Serving: Calories: 517; Saturated Fat: 6g; Cholesterol: 101mg; Sodium: 234mg; Calcium: 115mg; Carbohydrates: 32g; Protein: 42g

BEEF CHOW MEIN

Serves 4 | Prep time: 25 minutes | Cook time: 30 minutes

Asian-inspired food is thought to be packed with monosodium glutamate (MSG), a flavoring linked to headaches and other health concerns, but this homemade beef chow mein has no damaging additions—just piles of healthy vegetables and strips of juicy beef. The variety of ingredients includes all the nutrients recommended to manage fibromyalgia symptoms. Substitute chicken or pork for the beef without changing the nutrition profile extensively. This dish is delicious served over cauliflower rice.

BRAIN BOOSTER
DAIRY-FREE
GLUTEN-FREE
IMMUNE BOOSTER

1½ cups gluten-free, sodium-free beef broth

¼ cup coconut aminos

2 tablespoons xylitol

2 tablespoons arrowroot powder

1 tablespoon grated fresh ginger

Pinch red pepper flakes

2 tablespoons sesame oil

1 pound sliced beef striploin steak

2 cups sliced button mushrooms

3 celery stalks, sliced

2 carrots, sliced into thin disks

1 red bell pepper, thinly sliced

1 yellow bell pepper, thinly sliced

3 scallions, white and green parts, chopped

1 cup bean sprouts

2 tablespoons sesame seeds

1. In a small bowl, whisk the beef broth, coconut aminos, xylitol, arrowroot powder, ginger, and red pepper flakes. Set aside.

2. In a very large skillet or wok over medium-high heat, heat the sesame oil.

3. Add the beef and cook just until a little pink. Using a slotted spoon, transfer to a plate and set aside.

4. Return the skillet to the heat, and add the mushrooms, celery, carrots, red and yellow bell peppers, and scallions. Stir-fry for about 10 minutes, until the vegetables are crisp-tender.

5. Move the vegetables to the side of the skillet and pour in the sauce. Cook for about 3 minutes, stirring until the sauce is thick.

6. Toss the vegetables, reserved beef, and bean sprouts with the sauce for about 2 minutes, until heated through and coated. Serve topped with the sesame seeds.

Per Serving: Calories: 404; Saturated Fat: 6g; Cholesterol: 101mg; Sodium: 132mg; Calcium: 87mg; Carbohydrates: 16g; Protein: 40g

BEEF POT ROAST
WITH VEGETABLES

Serves 4 | Prep time: 20 minutes | Cook time: 1 hour, 10 minutes

Sunday roasts are a regular dish in many households because the meat and vegetables can be cooked together in one big roasting dish with minimal cleanup. Beef is a fantastic source of creatine protein, which can help reduce some of the muscle weakness and pain linked to fibromyalgia.

3 tablespoons extra-virgin olive oil

2 pounds beef pot roast

Himalayan salt or table salt, for seasoning

Freshly ground black pepper, for seasoning

3 carrots, cut into 1-inch chunks

2 sweet onions, cut into eight wedges

2 sweet potatoes, cut into large chunks

1 celeriac, peeled and cut into large chunks

3 garlic cloves, crushed

2 cups gluten-free, sodium-free beef broth

BRAIN BOOSTER
DAIRY-FREE
GLUTEN-FREE
IMMUNE BOOSTER
NUT-FREE
PALEO-FRIENDLY

1. Preheat the oven to 375°F.
2. In a large roasting pan over medium-high heat, heat the olive oil.
3. Season the beef generously all over with salt and pepper.
4. Add the beef to the pan, and cook for about 10 minutes, browning it on all sides. Transfer the meat to a plate and set aside.
5. Place one-fourth each of the carrots, onions, sweet potatoes, celeriac, and garlic in the roasting pan, and lay the beef on top of the vegetables. Arrange the remaining vegetables around the beef, and pour the beef broth into the pan.
6. Roast the beef for about 1 hour for medium, or to your desired doneness.
7. Let the beef rest for 10 minutes, slice, and serve with the vegetables.

Per Serving: Calories: 432; Saturated Fat: 4g; Cholesterol: 22mg; Sodium: 654mg; Calcium: 133mg; Carbohydrates: 48g; Protein: 19g

ITALIAN-STYLE MEATBALLS

Serves 4 | Prep time: 25 minutes | Cook time: 25 minutes

Meatballs are incredibly versatile: the perfect choice for appetizers, delicious smothered in sauce, excellent served alone as a main course, or an ideal snack tucked into lettuce wraps. The herbs used in this recipe create a unique flavor profile, but customize them to your liking for a different taste. Oregano is high in vitamin K, fiber, manganese, and iron. Manganese helps stabilize blood sugar and fight free radicals in the body. Iron increases oxygen flow to the muscles to fight fatigue and increase energy.

1½ pounds ground beef

1 sweet onion, chopped

½ cup almond flour

½ cup chopped fresh parsley leaves

2 tablespoons chopped fresh basil leaves

2 tablespoons chopped fresh oregano leaves

2 eggs

1 tablespoon minced garlic Himalayan salt or table salt, for seasoning

Freshly ground black pepper, for seasoning

BRAIN BOOSTER
DAIRY-FREE
GLUTEN-FREE
IMMUNE BOOSTER
PALEO-FRIENDLY

1. Preheat the oven to 350°F.
2. Line a rimmed baking sheet with aluminum foil.
3. In a large bowl, mix together the beef, onion, almond flour, parsley, basil, oregano, eggs, and garlic until very well mixed. Season with salt and pepper.
4. Using your hands, roll the mixture into golf ball-size meatballs and place them on the prepared sheet.
5. Bake for about 25 minutes until browned and cooked through. Serve.

SIMPLIFY IT: Meatballs freeze beautifully and can be placed in freezer bags either raw or cooked for later use. If you want to store them raw, place them on a baking sheet in the freezer until they are half frozen before transferring them to a bag.

Per Serving: Calories: 432; Saturated Fat: 5g; Cholesterol: 234mg; Sodium: 209mg; Calcium: 81mg; Carbohydrates: 6g; Protein: 56g

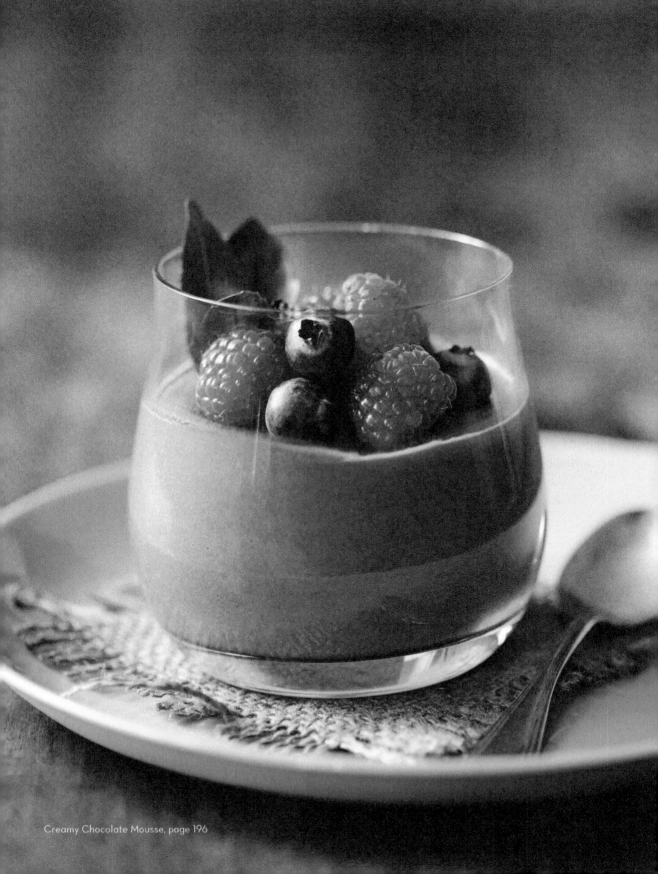

Creamy Chocolate Mousse, page 196

11
desserts

BLUEBERRY PANNA
COTTA 194

CITRUS-BERRY
AMBROSIA 195

CREAMY CHOCOLATE
MOUSSE 196

SWEET POTATO
PUDDING 197

LIME CHEESECAKE 198

BERRY BROWN BETTY 199

DARK CHOCOLATE
SHEET CAKE 200

BLUEBERRY PANNA COTTA

Serves 4 | Prep time: 20 minutes, plus 3 hours chilling time | Cook time: 10 minutes

Panna cotta *means "cooked cream," which is appropriate as this velvety smooth creation is made with heavy cream. Full-fat dairy, like the cream, is a smart addition to a fibromyalgia diet because healthy fats are needed to produce hormones that facilitate cell repair and effective brain function. Eating fats can also help you control food cravings and feel fuller longer, which can help you reach weight loss goals.*

¼ cup cold water

1 tablespoon gelatin

2 cups heavy (whipping) cream

1 cup unsweetened almond milk

¼ cup xylitol

2 teaspoons alcohol-free vanilla extract

2 cups fresh blueberries

BRAIN BOOSTER
GLUTEN-FREE
IMMUNE BOOSTER

1. Pour the water into a small bowl and sprinkle in the gelatin. Let it sit for 10 minutes.
2. In a large saucepan over medium heat, whisk the heavy cream, almond milk, xylitol, and vanilla. Heat until the liquid is scalded; do not boil. Remove the cream mixture from the heat.
3. Whisk in the gelatin mixture to blend. Pour the mixture into 4 serving dishes, and chill for about 3 hours until set.
4. Serve topped with blueberries.

COOKING TIP: If you want a vegetarian version of this dessert, substitute the same amount of powdered agar-agar for the gelatin. Make sure you purchase powdered agar-agar and not flaked, because you would have to use triple the amount of flaked product to get the same results.

Per Serving: Calories: 278; Saturated Fat: 11g; Cholesterol: 82mg; Sodium: 64mg; Calcium: 153mg; Carbohydrates: 15g; Protein: 5g

CITRUS-BERRY AMBROSIA

Serves 6 | Prep time: 20 minutes | Cook time: 0 minutes

Ambrosia is a tradition around Christmas time and is often taken to neighborhood gatherings because it is simple, easy to prepare, and delicious. This recipe is a variation of the original, leaving out the pineapple and maraschino cherries. The dish features inflammation-fighting coconut and almonds, healthy fats in the form of yogurt, and antioxidant-rich berries and oranges, and gives you a real boost of energy.

1 cup toasted slivered almonds

1 cup unsweetened toasted shredded coconut

1 cup plain, full-fat yogurt

2 tablespoons xylitol

1 teaspoon ground cinnamon

3 oranges, peeled and segmented

1 cup sliced fresh strawberries

1 cup fresh blueberries

BRAIN BOOSTER
GLUTEN-FREE
IMMUNE BOOSTER
VEGETARIAN

1. In a small bowl, stir together the almonds and coconut. Set aside.

2. In another small bowl, stir together the yogurt, xylitol, and cinnamon until blended.

3. In a medium bowl, toss the oranges, strawberries, and blueberries to mix.

4. Divide the fruit among 6 bowls, and top with the yogurt mixture.

5. Sprinkle the desserts with the almond-coconut mixture and serve.

Per Serving: Calories: 308; Saturated Fat: 10g; Cholesterol: 2mg; Sodium: 36mg; Calcium: 162mg; Carbohydrates: 27g; Protein: 9g

CREAMY CHOCOLATE MOUSSE

Serves 4 | Prep time: 20 minutes, plus 1 hour chilling time | Cook time: 0 minutes

This luscious, decadent mousse has a surprising hint of heat from the cayenne pepper. Rightly so, pairing chocolate and chile is a very popular combination because the chile deepens the delightful chocolate flavor. Both ingredients are powerful inflammation fighters and energy boosters, containing heaps of antioxidants and phytonutrients. The heavy cream adds appetite-suppressing healthy fats and hormone support.

2 cups heavy (whipping) cream

¼ cup xylitol

2 tablespoons cocoa powder

1 teaspoon alcohol-free vanilla extract

Pinch cayenne pepper

Pinch Himalayan salt or table salt

½ cup mixed fresh berries (optional)

GLUTEN-FREE
NUT-FREE
VEGETARIAN

1. In a large bowl, beat the heavy cream with an electric hand mixer until soft peaks form.
2. In a small bowl, stir together the xylitol, cocoa, vanilla, cayenne, and salt until well blended.
3. Beat the cocoa mixture into the whipped cream. Spoon the mousse into a serving bowl.
4. Refrigerate for 1 hour.
5. Serve garnished with berries (if using).

Per Serving: Calories: 226; Saturated Fat: 11g; Cholesterol: 82mg; Sodium: 82mg; Calcium: 43mg; Carbohydrates: 6g; Protein: 2g

SWEET POTATO PUDDING

Serves 4 | Prep time: 20 minutes, plus 1 hour chilling time | Cook time: 0 minutes

If you are a fan of pumpkin pie, you will love this warmly spiced creamy pudding. One of the most prevalent spices in this pretty dessert is cloves. Cloves are extremely high in antioxidants, including the flavonoids kaempferol and rhamnetin. They also contain a compound called eugenol that protects against inflammation by blocking the inflammation-causing enzyme COX-2. (COX-2 is also targeted by NSAIDS [nonsteroidal anti-inflammatory drugs], so this spice works in a similar fashion.)

2 cups coconut milk

1 cup mashed cooked sweet potato

¼ cup xylitol

1 teaspoon ground cinnamon

½ teaspoon ground ginger

Pinch ground cloves

¼ cup chopped pecans

BRAIN BOOSTER
DAIRY-FREE
GLUTEN-FREE
IMMUNE BOOSTER
VEGETARIAN

1. In a large bowl, whisk the coconut milk, sweet potato, xylitol, cinnamon, ginger, and cloves. Cover the bowl, and refrigerate the pudding for about 1 hour until chilled.

2. Serve the pudding topped with the pecans.

SIMPLIFY IT: When you make baked sweet potatoes as a side for a meal, throw in an extra one to use for this delectable dessert. Scoop the tender baked sweet potato flesh into a container and refrigerate it for up to 4 days.

Per Serving: Calories: 358; Saturated Fat: 25g; Cholesterol: 0mg; Sodium: 36mg; Calcium: 33mg; Carbohydrates: 21g; Protein: 4g

LIME CHEESECAKE

Serves 4 | Prep time: 20 minutes, plus 1 hour chilling time | Cook time: 0 minutes

Cheesecake is a delight. It is probably the first dessert people think of when considering the richest, most scrumptious treat they can splurge on. Cream cheese is a full-fat dairy product—that is important when considering the fat-soluble vitamins important for fibromyalgia, such as vitamins A, D, E, and K. Without fat, these nutrients are not available for the body to use for cell repair, fighting inflammation, and a host of other tasks.

¼ cup heavy (whipping) cream

1 tablespoon gelatin

8 ounces plain cream cheese,
   at room temperature

Zest of 1 lime

Juice of 1 lime

2 tablespoons xylitol

1 teaspoon alcohol-free vanilla extract

BRAIN BOOSTER

GLUTEN-FREE

IMMUNE BOOSTER

NUT-FREE

1. Pour the heavy cream into a small bowl, and sprinkle in the gelatin. Let it sit for 10 minutes.
2. Meanwhile, in a large bowl, beat the cream cheese with an electric hand mixer for about 5 minutes, until smooth and fluffy, scraping down the sides of the bowl.
3. Beat in the lime zest and juice, xylitol, and vanilla, scraping down the sides of the bowl at least once.
4. Beat in the gelatin mixture until well blended.
5. Spoon the mixture into 4 (4-ounce) ramekins, and refrigerate for about 1 hour until set. Serve.

Per Serving: Calories: 207; Saturated Fat: 11g; Cholesterol: 58mg; Sodium: 167mg; Calcium: 82mg; Carbohydrates: 9g; Protein: 6g

BERRY BROWN BETTY

Serves 4 | Prep time: 15 minutes | Cook time: 25 minutes

There are many names for this particular dessert including crumble, crisp, buckle, cobbler, and grunt. This is the "brown Betty" version because it does not include oats in the topping. Berries are uniformly rich in antioxidants, vitamins, and minerals, so if you are feeling creative, try different combinations, or in a pinch, go for a single type.

For the filling

2 cups fresh blueberries

2 cups fresh raspberries

1 tablespoon arrowroot powder

1 teaspoon ground cinnamon

½ teaspoon ground nutmeg

Pinch Himalayan salt or table salt

For the topping

¾ cup shredded unsweetened coconut

½ cup almond flour

1 tablespoon xylitol

¼ cup (½ stick) grass-fed butter,
   at room temperature

BRAIN BOOSTER
GLUTEN-FREE
IMMUNE BOOSTER
VEGETARIAN

Preheat the oven to 350°F.

To make the filling

1. In a medium bowl, stir together the blueberries, raspberries, arrowroot powder, cinnamon, nutmeg, and salt.
2. Spread the mixture into a 9-by-9-inch baking dish in an even layer.

To make the topping

1. In a medium bowl, stir together the coconut, almond flour, and xylitol until well mixed.
2. Stir in the butter until the mixture resembles coarse crumbs. Sprinkle the topping over the filling.
3. Bake for about 25 minutes until the topping is golden brown and the filling is bubbly. Serve.

Per Serving: Calories: 262; Saturated Fat: 10g; Cholesterol: 31mg; Sodium: 146mg; Calcium: 31mg; Carbohydrates: 23g; Protein: 4g

DARK CHOCOLATE SHEET CAKE

Serves 10 | Prep time: 15 minutes | Cook time: 40 minutes

Deep, dark fudge cake is the perfect choice for birthdays, holidays, and any day you need an energy boost or mood lift. Dark chocolate can improve mental clarity and concentration because it increases blood flow to the brain. The plethora of anti-oxidants in the cocoa reduces blood sugar, fights inflammation, and helps improve sleep quality. Who knew delicious could also be so beneficial for your health?

BRAIN BOOSTER
GLUTEN-FREE
IMMUNE BOOSTER
VEGETARIAN

1 cup (2 sticks) grass-fed butter, at room temperature, plus more for greasing the baking dish

1 cup xylitol

10 eggs

1 tablespoon alcohol-free vanilla extract

¾ cup coconut flour

½ cup cocoa powder

1 teaspoon baking soda

⅛ teaspoon Himalayan salt or table salt

1. Preheat the oven to 350°F.
2. Lightly grease a 9-by-13-inch baking dish with butter, and set it aside.
3. In a large bowl, beat together the butter and xylitol with an electric hand mixer until fluffy, scraping down the sides of the bowl at least once.
4. Beat in the eggs and vanilla until well blended, scraping down the sides of the bowl.
5. In a small bowl, stir together the coconut flour, cocoa, baking soda, and salt.
6. Add the dry ingredients to the wet ingredients, and beat until smooth. Pour the batter into the prepared dish.
7. Bake for about 40 minutes, until a knife inserted in the center comes out clean.
8. Remove the cake from the oven, and let it cool completely on a wire rack before serving.

Per Serving: Calories: 259; Saturated Fat: 14g; Cholesterol: 212mg; Sodium: 345mg; Calcium: 32mg; Carbohydrates: 8g; Protein: 7g

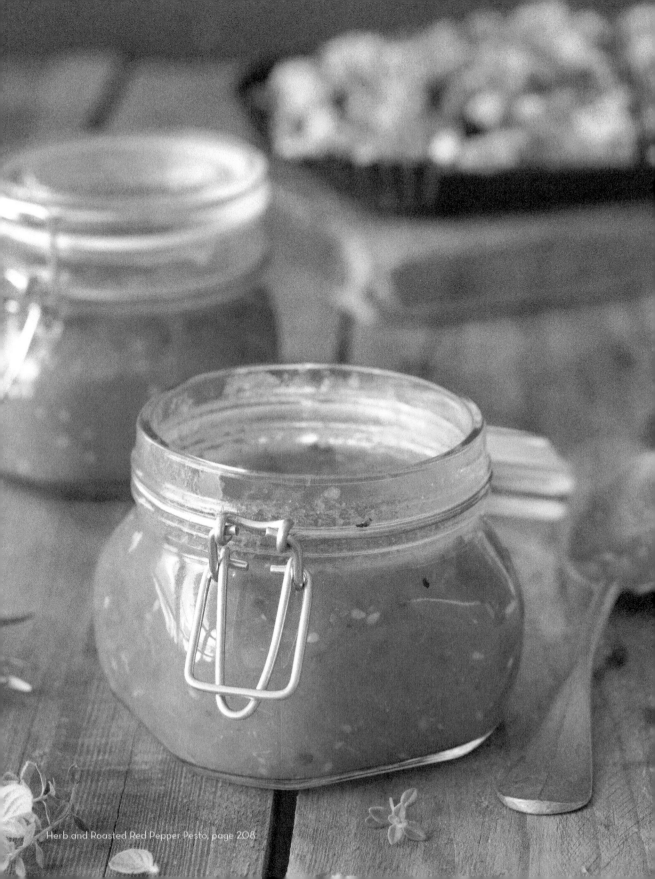

Herb and Roasted Red Pepper Pesto, page 208

12

staples: broths, sauces, & condiments

RICH BEEF BROTH   204

CHICKEN-VEGGIE
BROTH   206

HERB AND ROASTED
RED PEPPER PESTO   208

CHOCOLATE-ALMOND
SPREAD   209

CLASSIC GREMOLATA
SAUCE   210

SESAME-LEMON
DRESSING   211

VERSATILE BARBECUE
RUB   212

HOMEMADE ALMOND
MILK   213

CREAMY COCONUT
YOGURT   214

BLUEBERRY JAM   215

RICH BEEF BROTH

Makes 8 cups | Prep time: 15 minutes | Cook time: 6 hours, 30 minutes

You might think it does not matter what is put into the simmering water with beef bones when you make broth, but it is very important. Other ingredients, such as onion, garlic, celery, and carrots, called mirepoix *in professional kitchens, add flavor and nutrients to the finished broth. If you like the subtle taste of a certain herb like rosemary, marjoram, or sage, throw it into the pot.*

DAIRY-FREE
GLUTEN-FREE
IMMUNE BOOSTER
NUT-FREE
PALEO-FRIENDLY

2 pounds raw beef bones

1 sweet onion, quartered

4 garlic cloves, crushed

2 carrots, roughly chopped

2 celery stalks with their leaves, chopped

4 fresh thyme sprigs

1 teaspoon peppercorns

1. Preheat the oven to 375°F.
2. In a deep baking pan, combine the beef bones, onion, and garlic. Roast for 30 minutes.
3. Transfer the bones and veggies to a large stockpot over high heat, and add enough cold water to cover by about 4 inches. Bring to a boil, reduce the heat to low, and gently simmer for 4 hours, stirring every couple of hours.
4. Add the carrots, celery, thyme, and peppercorns. Return the broth to a boil, reduce the heat to low, and simmer for 2 hours more, stirring several times.
5. Remove the pot from the heat, and cool slightly.
6. Using tongs, remove any large bones. Strain the broth through a fine-mesh sieve and discard the solid bits.
7. Pour the broth into containers, and let it cool completely.
8. Refrigerate the broth in sealed containers for up to 5 days, or freeze for up to 3 months.

Per Serving (1 cup): Calories: 43; Saturated Fat: 0g; Cholesterol: 0mg; Sodium: 21mg; Calcium: 0mg; Carbohydrates: 1g; Protein: 3g

CHICKEN-VEGGIE BROTH

Makes 8 cups | Prep time: 15 minutes | Cook time: 6 hours, 30 minutes

Homemade broth is a fabulous ingredient to have on hand for all your recipes because you decide what goes into it and how it is flavored. Commercial broths are often packed with sodium and sometimes even sugar, which can play havoc with your health and diet goals. Because homemade broth keeps so well, it is easy to whip up a big batch and freeze in cup-size portions for future use.

DAIRY-FREE
GLUTEN-FREE
IMMUNE BOOSTER
NUT-FREE
PALEO-FRIENDLY

2 chicken carcasses

1 sweet onion, quartered

1 leek, well cleaned and chopped

4 garlic cloves, crushed

4 celery stalks with their leaves, cut into chunks

3 carrots, roughly chopped

4 fresh thyme sprigs

3 fresh parsley sprigs

1 teaspoon peppercorns

1. Preheat the oven to 375°F.
2. In a deep baking pan, combine the chicken carcasses, onion, leek, and garlic. Roast for 30 minutes.
3. Transfer the roasted carcasses and veggies to a large stockpot over high heat, and add enough cold water to cover by about 4 inches. Bring to a boil, reduce the heat to low, and gently simmer for 4 hours, stirring every couple of hours.
4. Add the celery, carrots, thyme, parsley, and peppercorns. Return the broth to a boil, reduce the heat to low, and simmer for 2 hours more, stirring several times.
5. Remove the pot from the heat, and cool slightly.
6. Using tongs, remove any large bones. Strain the broth through a fine-mesh sieve, and discard the solid bits.
7. Pour the broth into containers, and let it cool completely.
8. Refrigerate the broth in sealed containers for up to 5 days, or freeze for up to 3 months.

SIMPLIFY IT: Chicken carcasses can be stripped of meat and placed in the freezer in a sealed bag for several months. Save a couple to make this broth, placing them in the roasting dish right from the freezer.

Per Serving (1 cup): **Calories:** 32; **Saturated Fat:** 0g; **Cholesterol:** 0mg; **Sodium:** 56mg; **Calcium:** 0mg; **Carbohydrates:** 1g; **Protein:** 4g

HERB AND ROASTED
RED PEPPER PESTO

Makes 2 cups | Prep time: 10 minutes | Cook time: 0 minutes

Pesto is often made of herbs alone, so this lovely red sauce might be a nice surprise. Red bell peppers are a stellar source of vitamins C and E as well as carotenoids such as zeaxanthin and beta-carotene. When mixed with the allicin in garlic, healthy fats in pumpkin seeds, and antioxidant-rich basil, you have a fabulous choice for a sauce or dip to fight fibromyalgia symptoms.

3 roasted red bell peppers, seeded
½ cup fresh basil leaves
½ cup pumpkin seeds
3 garlic cloves
2 tablespoons chopped fresh parsley leaves
½ cup extra-virgin olive oil
Himalayan salt or table salt, for seasoning
Freshly ground black pepper, for seasoning

1. In a blender, combine the roasted peppers, basil, pumpkin seeds, garlic, and parsley. Pulse until finely chopped.
2. Add the olive oil, and blend until a thick paste forms.
3. Season the pesto with salt and pepper. Refrigerate in a sealed container for up to 1 week.

Per Serving (2 tablespoons): Calories: 94;
Saturated Fat: 1g; Cholesterol: 0mg; Sodium: 19mg;
Calcium: 83mg; Carbohydrates: 4g; Protein: 2g

BRAIN BOOSTER
DAIRY-FREE
GLUTEN-FREE
IMMUNE BOOSTER
NUT-FREE
PALEO-FRIENDLY
VEGETARIAN

CHOCOLATE-ALMOND SPREAD

Makes 2 cups | Prep time: 10 minutes | Cook time: 0 minutes

Do not confuse this delectable spread with the jars of similar products that populate the local grocery store shelves. This version is not packed with trans-fats and sugar, but instead contains healthy monounsaturated fats, fiber, iron, manganese, and copper. Cocoa can boost energy, fight inflammation, and boost blood flow to the muscles. Try different nuts, such as cashews or pecans, for delicious variations.

2 cups blanched almonds

½ cup coconut milk

¼ cup cocoa powder

2 tablespoons xylitol

2 teaspoons alcohol-free vanilla extract

Dash Himalayan salt or table salt

BRAIN BOOSTER
DAIRY-FREE
GLUTEN-FREE
IMMUNE BOOSTER
VEGETARIAN

1. In a food processor, pulse the almonds for about 10 minutes until they almost form a paste, scraping down the sides at least twice.
2. Add the coconut milk, cocoa, xylitol, vanilla, and salt. Blend until the mixture is very creamy and smooth.
3. Transfer to a sealed container, and refrigerate for up to 1 week.

Per Serving (2 tablespoons): **Calories:** 91; Saturated Fat: 2g; Cholesterol: 0mg; Sodium: 17mg; Calcium: 33mg; Carbohydrates: 4g; Protein: 3g

CLASSIC GREMOLATA SAUCE

Makes 1 cup | Prep time: 5 minutes | Cook time: 0 minutes

The base flavor in this pretty green sauce is parsley, but the lemon zest and juice are the stars, brightening all the other ingredients. Lemons are very high in vitamin C and flavonoids, reducing inflammation and fighting degenerative diseases. Scrub your lemons very well before zesting them, because they are often coated with wax applied to protect the fruit during transportation. You don't want to add that wax to your healthy sauce.

1 cup fresh parsley sprigs
2 tablespoons extra-virgin olive oil
1 tablespoon minced garlic
Zest of 1 lemon
Juice of 1 lemon
Himalayan salt or table salt, for seasoning

BRAIN BOOSTER
DAIRY-FREE
GLUTEN-FREE
IMMUNE BOOSTER
NUT-FREE
PALEO-FRIENDLY
VEGETARIAN

1. In a blender, combine the parsley, olive oil, garlic, lemon zest, and lemon juice. Pulse until finely chopped.
2. Season the sauce with salt. Refrigerate in a sealed container for up to 4 days.

COOKING TIP: This classic sauce can be made with any type of herb or even leafy dark greens or combinations of several types. Try different variations until you hit on a favorite.

Per Serving (2 tablespoons): Calories: 34; Saturated Fat: 1g; Cholesterol: 0mg; Sodium: 36mg; Calcium: 13mg; Carbohydrates: 1g; Protein: 0g

SESAME-LEMON DRESSING

Makes 1¼ cups | Prep time: 5 minutes | Cook time: 0 minutes

Tahini provides the rich sesame flavor in this delicious dressing along with many nutritional benefits. Sesame seeds, the base of tahini, are a fabulous source of magnesium, whose deficiency has been linked to fibromyalgia. Increasing your intake of magnesium can increase energy, reduce depression, and help fight both pain and tenderness in the muscles and joints. Magnesium is also crucial to balance calcium in the body to prevent muscle cramps and twitches.

1 cup coconut milk

¼ cup tahini

Juice of 1 lemon

½ teaspoon minced garlic

1 teaspoon minced fresh thyme leaves

Himalayan salt or table salt, for seasoning

1. In a small bowl, whisk the coconut milk, tahini, lemon juice, garlic, and thyme until well blended.
2. Season the dressing with salt. Refrigerate in a sealed container for up to 1 week.

Per Serving (2 tablespoons): Calories: 91; Saturated Fat: 5g; Cholesterol: 0mg; Sodium: 34mg; Calcium: 33mg; Carbohydrates: 3g; Protein: 2g

BRAIN BOOSTER

DAIRY-FREE

GLUTEN-FREE

IMMUNE BOOSTER

PALEO-FRIENDLY

VEGETARIAN

VERSATILE BARBECUE RUB

Makes ⅓ cup | Prep time: 5 minutes | Cook time: 0 minutes

Though black pepper shows up on almost every table right next to the salt, you may not realize it is an important addition to a healthy diet. Pepper is known as the "king of spices" and is an anti-inflammatory, antioxidant, and antibacterial. It also contains a chemical compound called piperine that is very effective, especially when the inflammation is in early stages. For the best flavor, use freshly ground pepper rather than an already ground product sitting in a jar.

2 tablespoons dried basil

2 tablespoons celery salt

1 tablespoon dried thyme

1 teaspoon freshly ground black pepper

1 teaspoon dried marjoram

1 teaspoon paprika

½ teaspoon ground coriander

1. In a small bowl, stir together the basil, celery salt, thyme, pepper, marjoram, paprika, and coriander until well blended.
2. Transfer the spice mixture to a sealed container, and store it in a cool dark place for up to 2 months.

Per Serving (1 tablespoon): Calories: 4; Saturated Fat: 0g; Cholesterol: 0mg; Sodium: 11mg; Calcium: 23mg; Carbohydrates: 1g; Protein: 0g

DAIRY-FREE
GLUTEN-FREE
IMMUNE BOOSTER
NUT-FREE
PALEO-FRIENDLY
VEGETARIAN

HOMEMADE ALMOND MILK

Makes 4 cups | Prep time: 15 minutes | Cook time: 0 minutes

Almonds are the seeds of the almond tree, and they are an excellent source of biotin, vitamins B₂ and E, manganese, copper, phosphorus, and magnesium. They help stabilize blood sugar, fight insomnia, and clear fibro fog, and are a fabulous source of monounsaturated fats—an effective part of a diet designed for weight loss (they make you feel full).

2 cups raw almonds

4 cups water

Pinch Himalayan salt or table salt

BRAIN BOOSTER
DAIRY-FREE
GLUTEN-FREE
IMMUNE BOOSTER
PALEO-FRIENDLY
VEGETARIAN

1. In a blender, combine the almonds, water, and salt. Blend for about 5 minutes, until the mixture is as smooth as possible.
2. Place fine-mesh cheesecloth over a pitcher, and pour the almond mixture through the cheesecloth.
3. Gather up the ends of the cloth, and squeeze out the liquid until the almond pulp is as dry as possible. Reserve the almond meal for other recipes.
4. Refrigerate the almond milk in a sealed container for up to 5 days.

Per Serving (1 cup): Calories: 40; Saturated Fat: 0g; Cholesterol: 0mg; Sodium: 180mg; Calcium: 200mg; Carbohydrates: 2g; Protein: 1g

CREAMY COCONUT YOGURT

Makes 2½ cups | Prep time: 5 minutes, plus 12 hours fermentation | Cook time: 0 minutes

Full-fat dairy products, such as plain yogurt, can be a healthy addition to your diet, but homemade coconut yogurt is a fabulous choice as well. Coconut contains medium chain triglycerides (MCTs) that go straight from the digestive tract to the liver where they become a quick source of energy. Coconut has multiple anti-inflammatory effects and can be an effective part of a weight loss strategy.

1 pound shredded unsweetened coconut

¼ cup coconut kefir

¼ cup heavy (whipping) cream

¼ cup freshly squeezed lemon juice

Pinch Himalayan salt or table salt

BRAIN BOOSTER
GLUTEN-FREE
IMMUNE BOOSTER
VEGETARIAN

1. In a blender, combine the coconut, coconut kefir, heavy cream, lemon juice, and salt. Process until very smooth and creamy. Transfer to a glass bowl and cover with fine-mesh cheesecloth.

2. Let the yogurt ferment at room temperature for at least 12 hours.

3. Stir the yogurt, and refrigerate it in a sealed container for up to 1 week.

A CLOSER LOOK: Kefir is a tart beverage that is rich in beneficial yeast and friendly probiotic bacteria. This ingredient is the yogurt's base because it cultures the other ingredients, creating the distinct tart flavor and thick texture.

Per Serving (¼ cup): Calories: 199; Saturated Fat: 16g; Cholesterol: 5mg; Sodium: 41mg; Calcium: 42mg; Carbohydrates: 8g; Protein: 2g

BLUEBERRY JAM

Makes 2 cups | Prep time: 5 minutes | Cook time: 10 minutes

This jam is not like supermarket jams, which have more sugar and preservatives in them than fruit. Blueberries are incredibly high in anti-inflammatory nutrients and phytonutrients and so can be a smart choice to add to your fibromyalgia-fighting diet to decrease the intensity of certain symptoms. The downside of a condiment bursting with fresh flavor and color is that it does not keep long, so enjoy it quickly!

2 cups fresh blueberries

2 tablespoons water

1 tablespoon xylitol

1 teaspoon alcohol-free vanilla extract

BRAIN BOOSTER
DAIRY-FREE
GLUTEN-FREE
IMMUNE BOOSTER
NUT-FREE
VEGETARIAN

1. In a medium saucepan over medium heat, combine the blueberries and water. Cook for about 10 minutes, stirring occasionally, until the blueberries burst and have a sauce-like texture. Remove from the heat.

2. Stir in the xylitol and vanilla. Transfer the jam to a container, and refrigerate it for about 1 hour until cool. Keep refrigerated in a sealed container for up to 1 week.

Per Serving (2 tablespoons): Calories: 12; Saturated Fat: 0g; Cholesterol: 0mg; Sodium: 0mg; Calcium: 0mg; Carbohydrates: 3g; Protein: 0g

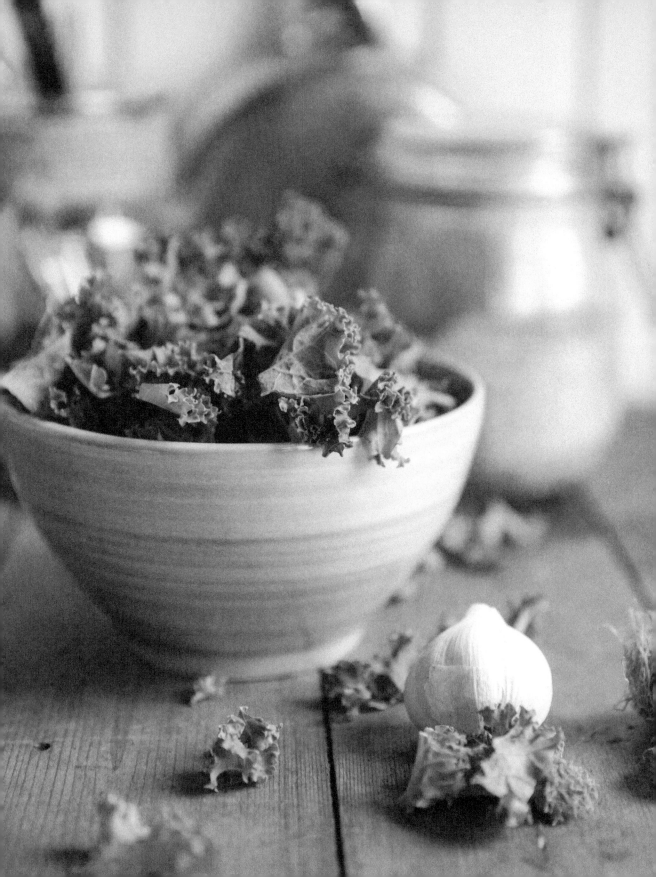

MEASUREMENT CONVERSIONS

Volume Equivalents (Liquid)

US STANDARD	US STANDARD (OUNCES)	METRIC (APPROXIMATE)
2 tablespoons	1 fl. oz.	30 mL
¼ cup	2 fl. oz.	60 mL
½ cup	4 fl. oz.	120 mL
1 cup	8 fl. oz.	240 mL
1½ cups	12 fl. oz.	355 mL
2 cups or 1 pint	16 fl. oz.	475 mL
4 cups or 1 quart	32 fl. oz.	1 L
1 gallon	128 fl. oz.	4 L

Oven Temperatures

FAHRENHEIT (F)	CELSIUS (C) (APPROXIMATE)
250°F	120°C
300°F	150°C
325°F	165°C
350°F	180°C
375°F	190°C
400°F	200°C
425°F	220°C
450°F	230°C

Volume Equivalents (Dry)

US STANDARD	METRIC (APPROXIMATE)
⅛ teaspoon	0.5 mL
¼ teaspoon	1 mL
½ teaspoon	2 mL
¾ teaspoon	4 mL
1 teaspoon	5 mL
1 tablespoon	15 mL
¼ cup	59 mL
⅓ cup	79 mL
½ cup	118 mL
⅔ cup	156 mL
¾ cup	177 mL
1 cup	235 mL
2 cups or 1 pint	475 mL
3 cups	700 mL
4 cups or 1 quart	1 L

Weight Equivalents

US STANDARD	METRIC (APPROXIMATE)
½ ounce	15 g
1 ounce	30 g
2 ounces	60 g
4 ounces	115 g
8 ounces	225 g
12 ounces	340 g
16 ounces or 1 pound	455 g

THE DIRTY DOZEN & THE CLEAN FIFTEEN

A nonprofit environmental watchdog organization called Environmental Working Group (EWG) looks at data supplied by the U.S. Department of Agriculture (USDA) and the Food and Drug Administration (FDA) about pesticide residues. Each year it compiles a list of the best and worst pesticide loads found in commercial crops. You can use these lists to decide which fruits and vegetables to buy organic to minimize your exposure to pesticides and which produce is considered safe enough to buy conventionally. This does not mean they are pesticide-free, though, so wash these fruits and vegetables thoroughly.

DIRTY DOZEN	CLEAN FIFTEEN
Apples	Asparagus
Celery	Avocados
Cherries	Cabbage
Grapes	Cantaloupes (domestic)
Nectarines	Cauliflower
Peaches	Eggplants
Pears	Grapefruits
Potatoes	Honeydew
Spinach	Kiwis
Strawberries	Mangoes
Sweet Bell Peppers	Onions
Tomatoes	Papayas
	Pineapples
In addition to the Dirty Dozen, the EWG added one type of produce contaminated with highly toxic organophosphate insecticides:	Sweet Corn
	Sweet peas (frozen)
Hot peppers	

RESOURCES

Seeking further information and support on fibromyalgia? Following are some of the best places to learn more.

Arthritis Foundation
www.arthritis.org

David Pearlmutter, MD
www.drperlmutter.com

FibroFix (Dr. David Brady)
www.fibrofix.com

Fibromyalgia Symptoms
www.fibromyalgia-symptoms.org

Food Sensitivities
www.nowleap.com
/the-patented-mediator-release-test-mrt/

Joe Cohen, SelfHacked
www.selfhacked.com

Mike Mutzel, High Intensity Health
www.highintensityhealth.com

PostureFit System
www.getposturefit.com

Trudy Scott, Food Mood Expert
www.everywomanover29.com

REFERENCES

Arthritis Foundation. "Arthritis Today Drug Guide." Accessed February 9, 2017. www.arthritis.org/living-with-arthritis/treatments/medication/drug-guide/.

Brady, David. "Fibromyalgia: Proper Diagnosis Is Half the Cure." *Townsend Letter: The Examiner of Alternative Medicine*. November 2016. Accessed February 9, 2017. www.townsendletter.com/Nov2016/fibro1116.html.

Carabotti, Marilia, Annunziata Scirocco, Maria Antonietta Maselli, and Carola Severi. "The Gut-Brain Axis: Interactions between Enteric Microbiota, Central, and Enteric Nervous Systems." *Annals of Gastroenterology: Quarterly Publication of the Hellenic Society of Gastroenterology* 28, no. 2 (April–June 2015): 203–209.

Cohen, Joe. "30 Natural Ways to Improve Mood by Increasing Our Opioids and Endorphins." *SelfHacked*. January 7, 2017. Accessed February 9, 2017. www.selfhacked.com/2014/09/10/why-the-ice-bucket-challenge-is-so-popular-it-functions-like-heroin/.

Cohen, Joe. "Brain Fog: The Causes, Treatment, and Cure." *SelfHacked*. February 08, 2017. Accessed February 9, 2017. www.selfhacked.com/2013/06/15/the-cause-of-brain-fog/.

FibromyalgiaSymptoms.org. "Men with Fibromyalgia." Accessed February 9, 2017. www.fibromyalgia-symptoms.org/fibromyalgia_relieve.html.

Fibromyalgia Treatment Group. "Three Symptoms of Fibromyalgia That Magnesium Could Alleviate." Accessed February 9, 2017. www.fibromyalgiatreatmentgroup.com/fibromyalgiatreatment/three-symptoms-of-fibromyalgia-that-magnesium-could-alleviate.

Gavi, M. B., D. V. Vassalo, F. T. Amaral, D. C. Macedo, P. L. Gava, E. M. Dantas, and V. Valim. "Strengthening Exercises Improve Symptoms and Quality of Life but Do Not Change Autonomic Modulation in Fibromyalgia: A Randomized Clinical Trial." *PLOS One* 9, no. 3 (March 20, 2014): e90767. doi:10.1371/journal.pone.0090767.

Healthline. "7 Foods That Could Boost Your Serotonin: Serotonin Diet." Accessed February 9, 2017. www.healthline.com/health/healthy-sleep/foods-that-could-boost-your-serotonin.

Juhl, John. "Fibromyalgia and the Serotonin Pathway." *Alternative Medicine Review* 3, no. 5 (1998): 367–75.

Konturek, P. C., T. Brzozowski, and S. J. Konturek. "Gut Clock: Implication of Circadian Rhythms in the Gastrointestinal Tract." *Journal of Physiology and Pharmacology* 62, no. 2 (April 2001): 139–50.

Landis, Carol A., Martha J. Lentz, James Rothermel, Stacy C. Riffle, Darla Chapman, Dedra Buchwald, and Joan L. F. Shaver. "Decreased Nocturnal Levels of Prolactin and Growth Hormone in Women with Fibromyalgia." *The Journal of Clinical Endocrinology and Metabolism* 86, no. 4 (2001): 1672–678. doi:10.1210/jcem.86.4.7427.

LifeExtension. "Pain (Chronic): Targeted Nutritional Intervention." LifeExtension: Health Protocols. Accessed February 9, 2017. www.lifeextension.com/Protocols/Health-Concerns/Chronic-Pain/Page-06.

Matallana, Lynne. "Women and Pain: A Focus on Fibromyalgia." National Fibromyalgia Association (NFA). Accessed February 9, 2017. www.fmaware.org/about-fibromyalgia/prevalence/women-fibro/.

Mayo Clinic Staff. "Selective Serotonin Reuptake Inhibitors (SSRIs)." Mayo Clinic. Accessed February 9, 2017. www.mayoclinic.org/diseases-conditions/depression/in-depth/ssris/art-20044825.

O'Connor, Patrick J., Matthew P. Herring, and Amanda Caravalho. "Mental Health Benefits of Strength Training in Adults." *American Journal of Lifestyle Medicine* 4, no. 5 (May 7, 2010): 377–96. doi:10.1177/1559827610368771.

Pasula, Mark. "The Patented Mediator Release Test (MRT): A Comprehensive Blood Test for Inflammation Caused by Food and Food-Chemical Sensitivities." *Townsend Letter* (January 2014).

Sangita Chakrabarty, MD, MSPH, and Roger Zoorob, MD, MPH. "Fibromyalgia." *American Family Physician* 76, no. 2 (July 15, 2007): 247–254.

Schaeffer, Juliann. "Color Me Healthy—Eating for a Rainbow of Benefits." *Today's Dietitian* 10, no. 11 (November 2008): 34. Accessed February 9, 2017. www.todaysdietitian.com/newarchives/110308p34.shtml.

Seneff, Stephanie, MD. "Sulfur Deficiency." *Wise Traditions in Food, Farming, and the Healing Arts*, the quarterly journal of the Weston A. Price Foundation. (July 2, 2011). Accessed February 9, 2017. www.westonaprice.org/health-topics/abcs-of-nutrition/sulfur-deficiency/.

Sivertsen, Børge, Tea Lallukka, Keith J. Petrie, Ólöf Anna Steingrímsdóttir, Audun Stubhaug, and Christopher Sivert Nielsen. "Sleep and Pain Sensitivity in Adults." *Pain* 156, no. 8 (August 2015): 1433–439. doi:10.1097/j.pain.0000000000000131.

University of Calgary. "Why Is Pain Important?" Accessed February 9, 2017. www.ucalgary.ca/pip369/mod7/tempain/impo.

Walling, Elizabeth. "Eight Natural Ways to Boost Serotonin and Mood." *NaturalNews*. May 27, 2009. Accessed February 9, 2017. www.naturalnews.com/026332_serotonin_natural_fat.html.

Walitt, Brian, Robert S. Katz, Martin J. Bergman, and Frederick Wolfe. "Three-Quarters of Persons in the US Population Reporting a Clinical Diagnosis of Fibromyalgia Do Not Satisfy Fibromyalgia Criteria: The 2012 National Health Interview Survey." *PLOS One* (June 9, 2016). doi:http://dx.doi.org/10.1371/journal.pone.0157235.

RECIPE INDEX

A

Acorn Squash Lamb
  Gratin, 184–185
Almond-Sesame Seed
  Balls, 107
Asian Spinach Salad with
  Almond Dressing, 92
Asparagus with Shallots, 125
Avocado-Chickpea
  Tabbouleh, 129
Avocado-Citrus Soup, 85
Avocado-Tangerine Salad, 97

B

Baked Sole with Parsley
  Pistou, 158
Baked Tilapia with
  Blueberry-Avocado
  Salsa, 163
Balsamic-Braised Onions, 117
Basil-Tomato Salad with Herb
  Vinaigrette, 93
Beef Chow Mein, 188–189
Beef Pot Roast with
  Vegetables, 190
Bell Pepper-Asparagus
  Frittata, 76
Berry Brown Betty, 199
Blueberry-Almond
  Scones, 108–109
Blueberry Jam, 215
Blueberry Panna Cotta, 194

C

Cajun Scallops, 139
Caramelized Onion and
  Spinach Omelet, 71
Chicken Breasts with
  Raspberry Sauce, 170–171
Chicken Cacciatore, 172
Chicken Chili Soup, 89
Chicken-Veggie
  Broth, 206–207
Chicken with Wild
  Mushrooms, 167
Chickpea Basil-Stuffed
  Peppers, 124
Chocolate-Almond
  Spread, 209
Chocolate-Pistachio Shake, 64
Chopped Veggie Bowl, 131
Cinnamon Cheesecake
  Smoothie, 67
Citrus-Berry Ambrosia, 195
Classic Gremolata Sauce, 210
Coconut Milk-Baked
  Catfish, 156
Coconut Milk-Braised
  Chicken, 173
Coconut Milk-Turmeric
  Smoothie, 68
Coconut-Tomato Seafood
  Curry, 148–149
Cold Cucumber-Dill Soup, 78
Creamy Chocolate
  Mousse, 196
Creamy Coconut Yogurt, 214
Creamy Saffron Chicken, 166
Creamy Summer Zoodles, 134
Crispy Baked Parsnip
  Fries, 104
Cucumber Green Smoothie, 65
Curried Cabbage Salad, 94
Curried Kohlrabi, 118–119

D

Dark Chocolate Sheet
  Cake, 200–201

E

Easy Chicken Pad
  Thai, 168–169

F

Fresh Summer Salad, 91

G

Garlic Shrimp and
  Vegetables, 140
Ginger-Coconut Cookies, 105
Gingered Asparagus, 121
Glorious Carrot Soup, 88
Golden Cottage
  Cheese-Topped Bass, 150
Grapefruit-Yogurt
  Smoothie, 69
Greek Fish Stew, 144–145

H

Harissa-Rubbed Bass, 151
Herb and Roasted Red Pepper
    Pesto, 208
Homemade Almond Milk, 213
Homemade Sauerkraut, 120

I

Italian-Style Meatballs, 191

K

Kale-Mixed Vegetable
    Salad, 98–99

L

Lamb-Vegetable Stew, 182–183
Lettuce Spring Rolls, 103
Lime Cheesecake, 198

M

Mediterranean Spaghetti
    Squash, 111
Mixed Nut Porridge, 70
Mussels in Coconut Broth, 138
Mustard-Crusted Venison, 181

N

Nut-Chili Crackers, 106

O

Open-Faced Egg Sandwiches
    on Kale, 78–79
Orange-Pistachio Bass, 147

P

Panfried Tilapia
    with Compound
    Butter, 152–153

Pesto-Kale Salad, 96
Pork Tenderloin with
    Caramelized Onions, 179
Portobello Mushroom–Baked
    Eggs, 128
Pretty Pickled
    Jalapeños, 112–113
Pumpkin, Turkey, and Swiss
    Chard Hash, 72

R

Radish and Chicken
    Salad-Stuffed Endive, 110
Radish and Egg Salad, 95
Refreshing Gazpacho, 82
Rich Beef Broth, 204–205
Roasted Bell Pepper
    Trout, 160–161
Roasted Cauliflower-Broccoli
    Soup, 87
Roasted Eggplant Dip, 102
Roasted Sole with Vegetables,
    Garlic, and Sunflower
    Seeds, 146
Roasted Trout with Fennel, 157
Roasted Vegetables with
    Thyme, 130
Roasted Venison Leg, 180

S

Sausage with Celeriac
    Latkes, 75
Scrambled Egg and Kale, 74
Sesame-Lemon Dressing, 211
Shrimp Egg Foo
    Young, 142–143
Simple Falafel, 126–127
Simple Pork Sausage, 77
Sole with Ginger-Wasabi
    Glaze, 162
Southwestern Cauliflower
    Rice, 116

Spice-Rubbed Flounder with
    Citrus Salsa, 154–155
Sweet Potato and Chickpea
    Sauté, 132–133
Sweet Potato-Brussels Sprouts
    Toss, 115
Sweet Potato Pudding, 197

T

Thai Coconut Milk Soup, 84
Thyme-Baked Artichokes, 114
Tomato-Baked Bass, 159
Tomato-Jalapeño Soup, 86
Traditional Herbed
    Meatloaf, 186
Trout-Pumpkin Patties, 141
Turkey Chili, 178
Turkey, Leek, and Pumpkin
    Casserole, 174
Turkey Shepherd's Pie, 176–177
Turkey Stroganoff, 175
Turkey-Zucchini Noodle
    Salad, 90

V

Vanilla-Kale Smoothie, 66
Veggie Breakfast Skillet, 73
Versatile Barbecue Rub, 212

W

Winter Vegetable Stew, 135

Z

Zucchini Pasta with Beef and
    Eggplant Sauce, 187

INDEX

A

Aflatoxins, 18
Alkaloids, 15
Allodynia, 7
Almond butter
Almond-Sesame Seed
Balls, 107
Asian Spinach Salad with
Almond Dressing, 92
Easy Chicken Pad
Thai, 168–169
Almond flour
Acorn Squash Lamb
Gratin, 184–185
Berry Brown Betty, 199
Blueberry-Almond
Scones, 108–109
Golden Cottage Cheese-
Topped Bass, 150
Italian-Style Meatballs, 191
Mixed Nut Porridge, 70
Nut-Chili Crackers, 106
Simple Falafel, 126–127
Traditional Herbed
Meatloaf, 186
Trout-Pumpkin Patties, 141
Almond milk
Blueberry Panna Cotta, 194
Cinnamon Cheesecake
Smoothie, 67
Coconut Milk-Turmeric
Smoothie, 68
Mixed Nut Porridge, 70
Vanilla-Kale Smoothie, 66

Almonds
Almond-Sesame Seed
Balls, 107
Asian Spinach Salad with
Almond Dressing, 92
Chocolate-Almond
Spread, 209
Citrus-Berry Ambrosia, 195
Coconut-Tomato Seafood
Curry, 148–149
Homemade Almond
Milk, 213
Animal products. *See also
specific*
organic, 15, 19
shopping for, 39
Anthocyanin, 15–17
Antioxidants, 9, 14–15
Anxiety, 7, 18, 44
Artichokes
Greek Fish Stew, 144–145
Pesto-Kale Salad, 96
Thyme-Baked Artichokes, 114
Asparagus
Asparagus with Shallots, 125
Bell Pepper-Asparagus
Frittata, 76
Garlic Shrimp and
Vegetables, 140
Gingered Asparagus, 121
Radish and Egg Salad, 95
Avocados
Avocado-Chickpea
Tabbouleh, 129
Avocado-Citrus Soup, 85
Avocado-Tangerine Salad, 97

Baked Tilapia with
Blueberry-Avocado
Salsa, 163
Chocolate-Pistachio
Shake, 64
Cold Cucumber-Dill Soup, 83
Creamy Summer
Zoodles, 134
Refreshing Gazpacho, 82
Vanilla-Kale Smoothie, 66

B

Bacon
Open-Faced Egg Sandwiches
on Kale, 78–79
Basil
Balsamic-Braised Onions, 117
Basil-Tomato Salad with
Herb Vinaigrette, 93
Bell Pepper-Asparagus
Frittata, 76
Chicken Cacciatore, 172
Chickpea Basil-Stuffed
Peppers, 124
Curried Kohlrabi, 118–119
Golden Cottage Cheese-
Topped Bass, 150
Herb and Roasted Red
Pepper Pesto, 208
Italian-Style Meatballs, 191
Kale-Mixed Vegetable
Salad, 98–99
Mediterranean Spaghetti
Squash, 111
Mussels in Coconut
Broth, 138

Basil *(continued)*
  Refreshing Gazpacho, 82
  Roasted Bell Pepper
    Trout, 160–161
  Simple Pork Sausage, 77
  Tomato-Baked Bass, 159
  Tomato-Jalapeño Soup, 86
  Traditional Herbed
    Meatloaf, 186
  Winter Vegetable Stew, 135
  Zucchini Pasta with Beef and
    Eggplant Sauce, 187
Bass
  Golden Cottage Cheese-
    Topped Bass, 150
  Harissa-Rubbed Bass, 151
  Orange-Pistachio Bass, 147
  Tomato-Baked Bass, 159
Bean sprouts
  Beef Chow Mein, 188–189
  Easy Chicken Pad
    Thai, 168–169
  Shrimp Egg Foo
    Young, 142–143
  Turkey-Zucchini Noodle
    Salad, 90
Beef
  Beef Chow Mein, 188–189
  Beef Pot Roast with
    Vegetables, 190
  Italian-Style Meatballs, 191
  Rich Beef Broth, 204–205
  Traditional Herbed
    Meatloaf, 186
  Zucchini Pasta with Beef and
    Eggplant Sauce, 187
Beets
  Pesto-Kale Salad, 96
  Roasted Sole with
    Vegetables, Garlic, and
    Sunflower Seeds, 146
Bell peppers
  Asian Spinach Salad with
    Almond Dressing, 92

Beef Chow Mein, 188–189
Bell Pepper-Asparagus
  Frittata, 76
Chicken Chili Soup, 89
Chickpea Basil-Stuffed
  Peppers, 124
Coconut-Tomato Seafood
  Curry, 148–149
Easy Chicken Pad
  Thai, 168–169
Fresh Summer Salad, 91
Garlic Shrimp and
  Vegetables, 140
Greek Fish Stew, 144–145
Harissa-Rubbed Bass, 151
Herb and Roasted Red
  Pepper Pesto, 208
Lettuce Spring Rolls, 103
Refreshing Gazpacho, 82
Roasted Bell Pepper
  Trout, 160–161
Scrambled Egg and Kale, 74
Tomato-Baked Bass, 159
Tomato-Jalapeño Soup, 86
Trout-Pumpkin Patties, 141
Turkey Chili, 178
Turkey-Zucchini Noodle
  Salad, 90
Veggie Breakfast Skillet, 73
Berries. *See specific*
Beta-carotene, 15
Blueberries
  about, 15
  Baked Tilapia with
    Blueberry-Avocado
    Salsa, 163
  Berry Brown Betty, 199
  Blueberry-Almond
    Scones, 108–109
  Blueberry Jam, 215
  Blueberry Panna Cotta, 194
  Citrus-Berry Ambrosia, 195
  Mixed Nut Porridge, 70

Bok choy
  Chicken Chili Soup, 89
  Coconut-Tomato Seafood
    Curry, 148–149
  Lamb-Vegetable
    Stew, 182–183
  Radish and Chicken
    Salad-Stuffed Endive, 110
Brain Booster recipes
  about, 45
  Acorn Squash Lamb
    Gratin, 184–185
  Almond-Sesame Seed
    Balls, 107
  Asian Spinach Salad with
    Almond Dressing, 92
  Asparagus with Shallots, 125
  Avocado-Chickpea
    Tabbouleh, 129
  Avocado-Citrus Soup, 85
  Avocado-Tangerine Salad, 97
  Baked Sole with Parsley
    Pistou, 158
  Baked Tilapia with
    Blueberry-Avocado
    Salsa, 163
  Basil-Tomato Salad with
    Herb Vinaigrette, 93
  Beef Chow Mein, 188–189
  Beef Pot Roast with
    Vegetables, 190
  Bell Pepper-Asparagus
    Frittata, 76
  Blueberry-Almond
    Scones, 108–109
  Blueberry Jam, 215
  Blueberry Panna Cotta, 194
  Cajun Scallops, 139
  Caramelized Onion and
    Spinach Omelet, 71
  Chicken Breasts with
    Raspberry Sauce, 170–171
  Chicken Cacciatore, 172
  Chicken Chili Soup, 89

Brain Booster recipes
    (continued)
Chicken with Wild
    Mushrooms, 167
Chocolate-Almond
    Spread, 209
Chocolate-Pistachio
    Shake, 64
Chopped Veggie Bowl, 131
Cinnamon Cheesecake
    Smoothie, 67
Citrus-Berry Ambrosia, 195
Classic Gremolata Sauce, 210
Coconut Milk-Baked
    Catfish, 156
Coconut Milk-Braised
    Chicken, 173
Coconut Milk-Turmeric
    Smoothie, 68
Coconut-Tomato Seafood
    Curry, 148–149
Cold Cucumber-Dill Soup, 83
Creamy Coconut Yogurt, 214
Creamy Saffron Chicken, 166
Creamy Summer
    Zoodles, 134
Cucumber Green
    Smoothie, 65
Curried Cabbage Salad, 94
Curried Kohlrabi, 118–119
Dark Chocolate Sheet
    Cake, 200–201
Easy Chicken Pad
    Thai, 168–169
Fresh Summer Salad, 91
Garlic Shrimp and
    Vegetables, 140
Gingered Asparagus, 121
Glorious Carrot Soup, 88
Golden Cottage
    Cheese-Topped Bass, 150
Grapefruit-Yogurt
    Smoothie, 69
Greek Fish Stew, 144–145
Harissa-Rubbed Bass, 151

Herb and Roasted Red
    Pepper Pesto, 208
Homemade Almond
    Milk, 213
Homemade Sauerkraut, 120
Italian-Style Meatballs, 191
Kale-Mixed Vegetable
    Salad, 98–99
Lamb-Vegetable
    Stew, 182–183
Lettuce Spring Rolls, 103
Lime Cheesecake, 198
Mediterranean Spaghetti
    Squash, 111
Mixed Nut Porridge, 70
Mussels in Coconut
    Broth, 138
Mustard-Crusted
    Venison, 181
Nut-Chili Crackers, 106
Open-Faced Egg Sandwiches
    on Kale, 78–79
Orange-Pistachio Bass, 147
Panfried Tilapia
    with Compound
    Butter, 152–153
Pesto-Kale Salad, 96
Pork Tenderloin with
    Caramelized Onions, 179
Portobello Mushroom–Baked
    Eggs, 128
Pretty Pickled
    Jalapeños, 112–113
Pumpkin, Turkey, and Swiss
    Chard Hash, 72
Radish and Chicken
    Salad-Stuffed Endive, 110
Radish and Egg Salad, 95
Refreshing Gazpacho, 82
Roasted Bell Pepper
    Trout, 160–161
Roasted Cauliflower-Broccoli
    Soup, 87
Roasted Eggplant Dip, 102

Roasted Sole with
    Vegetables, Garlic, and
    Sunflower Seeds, 146
Roasted Trout with
    Fennel, 157
Roasted Vegetables with
    Thyme, 130
Roasted Venison Leg, 180
Sausage with Celeriac
    Latkes, 75
Scrambled Egg and Kale, 74
Sesame-Lemon Dressing, 211
Shrimp Egg Foo
    Young, 142–143
Simple Falafel, 126–127
Sole with Ginger-Wasabi
    Glaze, 162
Southwestern Cauliflower
    Rice, 116
Spice-Rubbed Flounder with
    Citrus Salsa, 154–155
Sweet Potato and Chickpea
    Sauté, 132–133
Sweet Potato-Brussels
    Sprouts Toss, 115
Sweet Potato Pudding, 197
Thai Coconut Milk Soup, 84
Thyme-Baked Artichokes, 114
Tomato-Baked Bass, 159
Tomato-Jalapeño Soup, 86
Traditional Herbed
    Meatloaf, 186
Trout-Pumpkin Patties, 141
Turkey Chili, 178
Turkey, Leek, and Pumpkin
    Casserole, 174
Turkey Shepherd's Pie,
    176–177
Turkey Stroganoff, 175
Turkey-Zucchini Noodle
    Salad, 90
Vanilla-Kale Smoothie, 66
Veggie Breakfast Skillet, 73
Winter Vegetable Stew, 135
Zucchini Pasta with Beef and
    Eggplant Sauce, 187

Brain chemistry, 5
Broccoli
    Chopped Veggie Bowl, 131
    Kale-Mixed Vegetable
        Salad, 98–99
    Roasted Cauliflower-Broccoli
        Soup, 87
Brussels sprouts
    Sweet Potato-Brussels
        Sprouts Toss, 115

C

Cabbage
    Chopped Veggie Bowl, 131
    Curried Cabbage Salad, 94
    Homemade Sauerkraut, 120
    Lettuce Spring Rolls, 103
Carrots
    Asian Spinach Salad with
        Almond Dressing, 92
    Beef Chow Mein, 188–189
    Beef Pot Roast with
        Vegetables, 190
    Chicken Chili Soup, 89
    Chicken-Veggie
        Broth, 206–207
    Chopped Veggie Bowl, 131
    Coconut Milk-Turmeric
        Smoothie, 68
    Coconut-Tomato Seafood
        Curry, 148–149
    Curried Cabbage Salad, 94
    Easy Chicken Pad
        Thai, 168–169
    Fresh Summer Salad, 91
    Glorious Carrot Soup, 88
    Lamb-Vegetable
        Stew, 182–183
    Lettuce Spring Rolls, 103
    Rich Beef Broth, 204–205
    Roasted Sole with
        Vegetables, Garlic, and
        Sunflower Seeds, 146
    Roasted Trout with
        Fennel, 157

Roasted Vegetables with
    Thyme, 130
Sweet Potato and Chickpea
    Sauté, 132–133
Turkey Shepherd's
    Pie, 176–177
Turkey-Zucchini Noodle
    Salad, 90
Winter Vegetable Stew, 135
Cashews
    Baked Sole with Parsley
        Pistou, 158
    Curried Cabbage Salad, 94
    Easy Chicken Pad
        Thai, 168–169
    Mixed Nut Porridge, 70
    Mustard-Crusted
        Venison, 181
    Radish and Chicken
        Salad-Stuffed Endive, 110
Catfish
    Coconut Milk-Baked
        Catfish, 156
Cauliflower
    Asparagus with Shallots, 125
    Avocado-Chickpea
        Tabbouleh, 129
    Chopped Veggie Bowl, 131
    Coconut-Tomato Seafood
        Curry, 148–149
    Fresh Summer Salad, 91
    Garlic Shrimp and
        Vegetables, 140
    Kale-Mixed Vegetable
        Salad, 98–99
    Pesto-Kale Salad, 96
    Roasted Cauliflower-Broccoli
        Soup, 87
    Southwestern Cauliflower
        Rice, 116
    Turkey, Leek, and Pumpkin
        Casserole, 174
    Turkey Shepherd's
        Pie, 176–177
    Veggie Breakfast Skillet, 73

Celeriac
    Beef Pot Roast with
        Vegetables, 190
    Sausage with Celeriac
        Latkes, 75
    Sweet Potato and Chickpea
        Sauté, 132–133
    Winter Vegetable Stew, 135
Celery
    Acorn Squash Lamb
        Gratin, 184–185
    Beef Chow Mein, 188–189
    Chicken Chili Soup, 89
    Chicken-Veggie
        Broth, 206–207
    Chopped Veggie Bowl, 131
    Cold Cucumber-Dill Soup, 83
    Lamb-Vegetable
        Stew, 182–183
    Rich Beef Broth, 204–205
    Spice-Rubbed Flounder with
        Citrus Salsa, 154–155
    Turkey Shepherd's
        Pie, 176–177
Chicken
    Avocado-Citrus Soup, 85
    Chicken Breasts with
        Raspberry Sauce, 170–171
    Chicken Cacciatore, 172
    Chicken Chili Soup, 89
    Chicken-Veggie
        Broth, 206–207
    Chicken with Wild
        Mushrooms, 167
    Coconut Milk-Braised
        Chicken, 173
    Creamy Saffron Chicken, 166
    Easy Chicken Pad
        Thai, 168–169
    Fresh Summer Salad, 91
    Radish and Chicken
        Salad-Stuffed Endive, 110
Chickpeas
    Avocado-Chickpea
        Tabbouleh, 129

Chickpeas (continued)
Chickpea Basil-Stuffed
Peppers, 124
Simple Falafel, 126–127
Sweet Potato and Chickpea
Sauté, 132–133
Chocolate. See Cocoa powder
Chronic fatigue, 7–8, 19
Chronic pain, 7–8, 42–43
Cilantro
Asian Spinach Salad with
Almond Dressing, 92
Avocado-Citrus Soup, 85
Baked Tilapia with
Blueberry-Avocado
Salsa, 163
Chicken Chili Soup, 89
Coconut Milk-Baked
Catfish, 156
Coconut Milk-Braised
Chicken, 173
Creamy Summer
Zoodles, 134
Lettuce Spring Rolls, 103
Refreshing Gazpacho, 82
Roasted Venison Leg, 180
Sole with Ginger-Wasabi
Glaze, 162
Southwestern Cauliflower
Rice, 116
Spice-Rubbed Flounder with
Citrus Salsa, 154–155
Thai Coconut Milk Soup, 84
Turkey-Zucchini Noodle
Salad, 90
Circadian rhythm, 8
Cocoa powder
Chocolate-Almond
Spread, 209
Chocolate-Pistachio
Shake, 64
Creamy Chocolate
Mousse, 196
Dark Chocolate Sheet
Cake, 200–201

Coconut
Berry Brown Betty, 199
Citrus-Berry Ambrosia, 195
Creamy Coconut Yogurt, 214
Thai Coconut Milk Soup, 84
Coconut flour
Dark Chocolate Sheet
Cake, 200–201
Ginger-Coconut Cookies, 105
Mixed Nut Porridge, 70
Coconut milk
Chocolate-Almond
Spread, 209
Chocolate-Pistachio
Shake, 64
Coconut Milk-Baked
Catfish, 156
Coconut Milk-Braised
Chicken, 173
Coconut Milk-Turmeric
Smoothie, 68
Coconut-Tomato Seafood
Curry, 148–149
Cucumber Green
Smoothie, 65
Grapefruit-Yogurt
Smoothie, 69
Mussels in Coconut
Broth, 138
Sesame-Lemon Dressing, 211
Sweet Potato Pudding, 197
Thai Coconut Milk Soup, 84
Cognitive dysfunction, 9, 18
Cottage cheese
Chickpea Basil-Stuffed
Peppers, 124
Golden Cottage
Cheese-Topped Bass, 150
Veggie Breakfast Skillet, 73
Cream cheese
Acorn Squash Lamb
Gratin, 184–185
Cinnamon Cheesecake
Smoothie, 67
Lime Cheesecake, 198

Cucumbers
Avocado-Chickpea
Tabbouleh, 129
Baked Tilapia with
Blueberry-Avocado
Salsa, 163
Cold Cucumber-Dill Soup, 83
Cucumber Green
Smoothie, 65
Kale-Mixed Vegetable
Salad, 98–99
Lettuce Spring Rolls, 103
Refreshing Gazpacho, 82

D

Dairy-Free recipes
about, 45
Almond-Sesame Seed
Balls, 107
Asian Spinach Salad with
Almond Dressing, 92
Avocado-Chickpea
Tabbouleh, 129
Avocado-Tangerine Salad, 97
Baked Sole with Parsley
Pistou, 158
Baked Tilapia with
Blueberry-Avocado
Salsa, 163
Balsamic-Braised Onions, 117
Beef Chow Mein, 188–189
Beef Pot Roast with
Vegetables, 190
Blueberry Jam, 215
Chicken Breasts with
Raspberry Sauce, 170–171
Chicken Cacciatore, 172
Chicken-Veggie
Broth, 206–207
Chocolate-Almond
Spread, 209
Chocolate-Pistachio
Shake, 64
Chopped Veggie Bowl, 131

Dairy-Free recipes *(continued)*
  Classic Gremolata Sauce, 210
  Coconut Milk-Turmeric
    Smoothie, 68
  Coconut-Tomato Seafood
    Curry, 148–149
  Cold Cucumber-Dill Soup, 83
  Crispy Baked Parsnip
    Fries, 104
  Cucumber Green
    Smoothie, 65
  Curried Kohlrabi, 118–119
  Easy Chicken Pad
    Thai, 168–169
  Fresh Summer Salad, 91
  Greek Fish Stew, 144–145
  Harissa-Rubbed Bass, 151
  Herb and Roasted Red
    Pepper Pesto, 208
  Homemade Almond
    Milk, 213
  Homemade Sauerkraut, 120
  Italian-Style Meatballs, 191
  Kale-Mixed Vegetable
    Salad, 98–99
  Lamb-Vegetable
    Stew, 182–183
  Lettuce Spring Rolls, 103
  Mediterranean Spaghetti
    Squash, 111
  Mussels in Coconut
    Broth, 138
  Mustard-Crusted
    Venison, 181
  Nut-Chili Crackers, 106
  Open-Faced Egg Sandwiches
    on Kale, 78–79
  Pesto-Kale Salad, 96
  Portobello Mushroom–Baked
    Eggs, 128
  Pretty Pickled Jalapeños,
    112–113
  Pumpkin, Turkey, and Swiss
    Chard Hash, 72

  Rich Beef Broth, 204–205
  Roasted Bell Pepper
    Trout, 160–161
  Roasted Eggplant Dip, 102
  Roasted Sole with
    Vegetables, Garlic, and
    Sunflower Seeds, 146
  Roasted Trout with
    Fennel, 157
  Roasted Vegetables with
    Thyme, 130
  Roasted Venison Leg, 180
  Sesame-Lemon Dressing, 211
  Shrimp Egg Foo
    Young, 142–143
  Simple Falafel, 126–127
  Simple Pork Sausage, 77
  Sole with Ginger-Wasabi
    Glaze, 162
  Southwestern Cauliflower
    Rice, 116
  Spice-Rubbed Flounder with
    Citrus Salsa, 154–155
  Sweet Potato and Chickpea
    Sauté, 132–133
  Sweet Potato-Brussels
    Sprouts Toss, 115
  Sweet Potato Pudding, 197
  Thai Coconut Milk Soup, 84
  Tomato-Baked Bass, 159
  Tomato-Jalapeño Soup, 86
  Trout-Pumpkin Patties, 141
  Turkey, Leek, and Pumpkin
    Casserole, 174
  Turkey-Zucchini Noodle
    Salad, 90
  Vanilla-Kale Smoothie, 66
  Versatile Barbecue Rub, 212
  Zucchini Pasta with Beef and
    Eggplant Sauce, 187
Digestive tract, 3–4, 8
Dill
  Cold Cucumber-Dill Soup, 83
  Roasted Trout with
    Fennel, 157

E
Eating your colors, 14–15
Edamame
  Creamy Summer
    Zoodles, 134
Eggplant
  Roasted Eggplant Dip, 102
  Zucchini Pasta with Beef and
    Eggplant Sauce, 187
Eggs
  Bell Pepper-Asparagus
    Frittata, 76
  Caramelized Onion and
    Spinach Omelet, 71
  Dark Chocolate Sheet
    Cake, 200–201
  Open-Faced Egg Sandwiches
    on Kale, 78–79
  Portobello Mushroom–Baked
    Eggs, 128
  Radish and Egg Salad, 95
  Scrambled Egg and Kale, 74
  Shrimp Egg Foo
    Young, 142–143
  Veggie Breakfast Skillet, 73
Elimination diets, 27–28
Endive
  Radish and Chicken
    Salad-Stuffed Endive, 110
Equipment, 39–41
Estrogen, 5–7
Exercise, 18–21

F
Fatigue, chronic, 8, 19
Fennel
  Cold Cucumber-Dill Soup, 83
  Roasted Trout with
    Fennel, 157
Fibro fog, 9, 18
Fibromites, 7
Fibromyalgia
  about, 3–4
  causes of, 4–7

exercise and, 18–21

signs and symptoms, 7–9

and sleep habits, 10

symptom tracking, 30–33, 44

Fibromyalgia diet

eating clean and, 13–15, 18

eliminating foods, 27–28

equipment for, 39–41

fighting brain fog meal
plan, 54–56

gaining energy meal
plan, 51–53

getting started, 25–26

pain management meal
plan, 48–50

pantry staples, 36–38

promoting healthy digestion
meal plan, 57–59

reintroducing foods, 28–30

shopping guide, 38–39

symptom tracking, 30–33, 44

tips and tricks for
success, 43–45

what to expect, 41–43

Fish. *See* Bass; Catfish;
Flounder; Sole; Tilapia;
Trout; Whitefish

Flavonoids, 15

Flaxseed

Coconut Milk-Turmeric
Smoothie, 68

Mixed Nut Porridge, 70

Flounder

Spice-Rubbed Flounder with
Citrus Salsa, 154–155

Food cravings, 44

Foods

to avoid, 14

eating your colors, 14–15

to enjoy, 14

and medications, vitamins,
and minerals, 16–17

organic, 15, 18

pantry staples, 36–38

shopping guide, 38–39

Free radicals, 9

Fruits. *See also specific*
shopping for, 38–39

G

Garlic

Garlic Shrimp and
Vegetables, 140

Herb and Roasted Red
Pepper Pesto, 208

Roasted Sole with
Vegetables, Garlic, and
Sunflower Seeds, 146

Trout-Pumpkin Patties, 141

Gastrointestinal (GI)
tract, 3–4, 8

Gender, and fibromyalgia, 6

Genetics, 5

Ginger

Asian Spinach Salad with
Almond Dressing, 92

Avocado-Tangerine Salad, 97

Beef Chow Mein, 188–189

Chicken Chili Soup, 89

Chopped Veggie Bowl, 131

Coconut Milk-Baked
Catfish, 156

Coconut Milk-Braised
Chicken, 173

Coconut-Tomato Seafood
Curry, 148–149

Cucumber Green
Smoothie, 65

Easy Chicken Pad
Thai, 168–169

Ginger-Coconut Cookies, 105

Gingered Asparagus, 121

Mussels in Coconut
Broth, 138

Shrimp Egg Foo
Young, 142–143

Sole with Ginger-Wasabi
Glaze, 162

Turkey-Zucchini Noodle
Salad, 90

Gluten-Free recipes

about, 45

Acorn Squash Lamb
Gratin, 184–185

Almond-Sesame Seed
Balls, 107

Asian Spinach Salad with
Almond Dressing, 92

Asparagus with Shallots, 125

Avocado-Chickpea
Tabbouleh, 129

Avocado-Citrus Soup, 85

Avocado-Tangerine Salad, 97

Baked Sole with Parsley
Pistou, 158

Baked Tilapia with
Blueberry-Avocado
Salsa, 163

Balsamic-Braised Onions, 117

Basil-Tomato Salad with
Herb Vinaigrette, 93

Beef Chow Mein, 188–189

Beef Pot Roast with
Vegetables, 190

Bell Pepper-Asparagus
Frittata, 76

Blueberry-Almond
Scones, 108–109

Blueberry Jam, 215

Blueberry Panna Cotta, 194

Cajun Scallops, 139

Caramelized Onion and
Spinach Omelet, 71

Chicken Breasts with
Raspberry Sauce, 170–171

Chicken Cacciatore, 172

Chicken Chili Soup, 89

Chicken-Veggie
Broth, 206–207

Chicken with Wild
Mushrooms, 167

Chickpea Basil-Stuffed
Peppers, 124

Gluten-Free recipes
    (continued)
Chocolate-Almond
    Spread, 209
Chocolate-Pistachio
    Shake, 64
Chopped Veggie Bowl, 131
Cinnamon Cheesecake
    Smoothie, 67
Citrus-Berry Ambrosia, 195
Classic Gremolata Sauce, 210
Coconut Milk-Baked
    Catfish, 156
Coconut Milk-Braised
    Chicken, 173
Coconut Milk-Turmeric
    Smoothie, 68
Coconut-Tomato Seafood
    Curry, 148–149
Cold Cucumber-Dill Soup, 83
Creamy Chocolate
    Mousse, 196
Creamy Coconut Yogurt, 214
Creamy Saffron Chicken, 166
Creamy Summer
    Zoodles, 134
Crispy Baked Parsnip
    Fries, 104
Cucumber Green
    Smoothie, 65
Curried Cabbage Salad, 94
Curried Kohlrabi, 118–119
Dark Chocolate Sheet
    Cake, 200–201
Easy Chicken Pad
    Thai, 168–169
Fresh Summer Salad, 91
Garlic Shrimp and
    Vegetables, 140
Ginger-Coconut Cookies, 105
Gingered Asparagus, 121
Glorious Carrot Soup, 88
Golden Cottage
    Cheese-Topped Bass, 150

Grapefruit-Yogurt
    Smoothie, 69
Greek Fish Stew, 144–145
Harissa-Rubbed Bass, 151
Herb and Roasted Red
    Pepper Pesto, 208
Homemade Almond
    Milk, 213
Homemade Sauerkraut, 120
Italian-Style Meatballs, 191
Kale-Mixed Vegetable
    Salad, 98–99
Lamb-Vegetable
    Stew, 182–183
Lettuce Spring Rolls, 103
Lime Cheesecake, 198
Mediterranean Spaghetti
    Squash, 111
Mixed Nut Porridge, 70
Mussels in Coconut
    Broth, 138
Mustard-Crusted
    Venison, 181
Nut-Chili Crackers, 106
Open-Faced Egg Sandwiches
    on Kale, 78–79
Orange-Pistachio Bass, 147
Panfried Tilapia with
    Compound Butter,
    152–153
Pesto-Kale Salad, 96
Pork Tenderloin with
    Caramelized Onions, 179
Portobello Mushroom–Baked
    Eggs, 128
Pretty Pickled
    Jalapeños, 112–113
Pumpkin, Turkey, and Swiss
    Chard Hash, 72
Radish and Chicken
    Salad-Stuffed Endive, 110
Radish and Egg Salad, 95
Refreshing Gazpacho, 82
Rich Beef Broth, 204–205

Roasted Bell Pepper
    Trout, 160–161
Roasted Cauliflower-Broccoli
    Soup, 87
Roasted Eggplant Dip, 102
Roasted Sole with
    Vegetables, Garlic, and
    Sunflower Seeds, 146
Roasted Trout with
    Fennel, 157
Roasted Vegetables with
    Thyme, 130
Roasted Venison Leg, 180
Sausage with Celeriac
    Latkes, 75
Scrambled Egg and Kale, 74
Sesame-Lemon Dressing, 211
Shrimp Egg Foo
    Young, 142–143
Simple Falafel, 126–127
Simple Pork Sausage, 77
Sole with Ginger-Wasabi
    Glaze, 162
Southwestern Cauliflower
    Rice, 116
Spice-Rubbed Flounder with
    Citrus Salsa, 154–155
Sweet Potato and Chickpea
    Sauté, 132–133
Sweet Potato-Brussels
    Sprouts Toss, 115
Sweet Potato Pudding, 197
Thai Coconut Milk Soup, 84
Thyme-Baked Artichokes, 114
Tomato-Baked Bass, 159
Tomato-Jalapeño Soup, 86
Traditional Herbed
    Meatloaf, 186
Trout-Pumpkin Patties, 141
Turkey Chili, 178
Turkey, Leek, and Pumpkin
    Casserole, 174
Turkey Shepherd's
    Pie, 176–177
Turkey Stroganoff, 175

Gluten-Free recipes
(continued)
Turkey-Zucchini Noodle
Salad, 90
Vanilla-Kale Smoothie, 66
Veggie Breakfast Skillet, 73
Versatile Barbecue Rub, 212
Winter Vegetable Stew, 135
Zucchini Pasta with Beef and
Eggplant Sauce, 187
Grapefruit
Grapefruit-Yogurt
Smoothie, 69
Spice-Rubbed Flounder with
Citrus Salsa, 154–155
Gut-brain axis, 4
Gut health, 4, 57

H

Hazelnuts
Chopped Veggie Bowl, 131
Hormonal imbalance, 5–7
Hydration, 45

I

Immune Booster recipes
about, 45
Acorn Squash Lamb
Gratin, 184–185
Almond-Sesame Seed
Balls, 107
Asian Spinach Salad with
Almond Dressing, 92
Asparagus with Shallots, 125
Avocado-Chickpea
Tabbouleh, 129
Avocado-Citrus Soup, 85
Avocado-Tangerine Salad, 97
Baked Sole with Parsley
Pistou, 158
Baked Tilapia with
Blueberry-Avocado
Salsa, 163

Balsamic-Braised Onions, 117
Basil-Tomato Salad with
Herb Vinaigrette, 93
Beef Chow Mein, 188–189
Beef Pot Roast with
Vegetables, 190
Bell Pepper-Asparagus
Frittata, 76
Blueberry-Almond
Scones, 108–109
Blueberry Jam, 215
Blueberry Panna Cotta, 194
Cajun Scallops, 139
Caramelized Onion and
Spinach Omelet, 71
Chicken Breasts with
Raspberry Sauce, 170–171
Chicken Cacciatore, 172
Chicken Chili Soup, 89
Chicken-Veggie
Broth, 206–207
Chicken with Wild
Mushrooms, 167
Chickpea Basil-Stuffed
Peppers, 124
Chocolate-Almond
Spread, 209
Chocolate-Pistachio
Shake, 64
Chopped Veggie Bowl, 131
Cinnamon Cheesecake
Smoothie, 67
Citrus-Berry Ambrosia, 195
Classic Gremolata Sauce, 210
Coconut Milk-Baked
Catfish, 156
Coconut Milk-Braised
Chicken, 173
Coconut Milk-Turmeric
Smoothie, 68
Coconut-Tomato Seafood
Curry, 148–149
Cold Cucumber-Dill Soup, 83
Creamy Coconut Yogurt, 214
Creamy Saffron Chicken, 166

Creamy Summer
Zoodles, 134
Crispy Baked Parsnip
Fries, 104
Cucumber Green
Smoothie, 65
Curried Cabbage Salad, 94
Curried Kohlrabi, 118–119
Dark Chocolate Sheet
Cake, 200–201
Easy Chicken Pad
Thai, 168–169
Fresh Summer Salad, 91
Garlic Shrimp and
Vegetables, 140
Ginger-Coconut Cookies, 105
Gingered Asparagus, 121
Glorious Carrot Soup, 88
Golden Cottage
Cheese-Topped Bass, 150
Grapefruit-Yogurt
Smoothie, 69
Greek Fish Stew, 144–145
Harissa-Rubbed Bass, 151
Herb and Roasted Red
Pepper Pesto, 208
Homemade Almond
Milk, 213
Homemade Sauerkraut, 120
Italian-Style Meatballs, 191
Kale-Mixed Vegetable
Salad, 98–99
Lamb-Vegetable
Stew, 182–183
Lettuce Spring Rolls, 103
Lime Cheesecake, 198
Mediterranean Spaghetti
Squash, 111
Mixed Nut Porridge, 70
Mussels in Coconut
Broth, 138
Mustard-Crusted
Venison, 181
Nut-Chili Crackers, 106

Immune Booster recipes
    (continued)
    Open-Faced Egg Sandwiches
        on Kale, 78–79
    Orange-Pistachio Bass, 147
    Panfried Tilapia with
        Compound Butter,
        152–153
    Pesto-Kale Salad, 96
    Pork Tenderloin with
        Caramelized Onions, 179
    Portobello Mushroom–Baked
        Eggs, 128
    Pretty Pickled
        Jalapeños, 112–113
    Pumpkin, Turkey, and Swiss
        Chard Hash, 72
    Radish and Chicken
        Salad-Stuffed Endive, 110
    Radish and Egg Salad, 95
    Refreshing Gazpacho, 82
    Rich Beef Broth, 204–205
    Roasted Bell Pepper
        Trout, 160–161
    Roasted Cauliflower-Broccoli
        Soup, 87
    Roasted Eggplant Dip, 102
    Roasted Sole with
        Vegetables, Garlic, and
        Sunflower Seeds, 146
    Roasted Trout with
        Fennel, 157
    Roasted Vegetables with
        Thyme, 130
    Roasted Venison Leg, 180
    Sausage with Celeriac
        Latkes, 75
    Scrambled Egg and Kale, 74
    Sesame-Lemon Dressing, 211
    Shrimp Egg Foo
        Young, 142–143
    Simple Falafel, 126–127
    Simple Pork Sausage, 77
    Sole with Ginger-Wasabi
        Glaze, 162
    Southwestern Cauliflower
        Rice, 116
    Spice-Rubbed Flounder with
        Citrus Salsa, 154–155
    Sweet Potato and Chickpea
        Sauté, 132–133
    Sweet Potato-Brussels
        Sprouts Toss, 115
    Sweet Potato Pudding, 197
    Thai Coconut Milk Soup, 84
    Thyme-Baked Artichokes, 114
    Tomato-Baked Bass, 159
    Tomato-Jalapeño Soup, 86
    Traditional Herbed
        Meatloaf, 186
    Trout-Pumpkin Patties, 141
    Turkey Chili, 178
    Turkey, Leek, and Pumpkin
        Casserole, 174
    Turkey Shepherd's
        Pie, 176–177
    Turkey Stroganoff, 175
    Turkey-Zucchini Noodle
        Salad, 90
    Vanilla-Kale Smoothie, 66
    Veggie Breakfast Skillet, 73
    Versatile Barbecue Rub, 212
    Winter Vegetable Stew, 135
    Zucchini Pasta with Beef and
        Eggplant Sauce, 187
Immune system, 3–4, 28
Impaired cognition, 9, 18
Inflammation, 4, 9, 15, 28
Ingredients
    foods to avoid, 14
    foods to enjoy, 14
    meal plans, 49–50, 52–53,
        55–56, 58–59
    pantry staples, 36–38
    shopping guide, 38–39
Insulin, 5
Intestinal permeability, 4

J
Jalapeño peppers
    Avocado-Citrus Soup, 85
    Chicken Chili Soup, 89
    Pretty Pickled
        Jalapeños, 112–113
    Refreshing Gazpacho, 82
    Southwestern Cauliflower
        Rice, 116
    Tomato-Jalapeño Soup, 86
Jicama
    Asian Spinach Salad with
        Almond Dressing, 92

K
Kale
    Asian Spinach Salad with
        Almond Dressing, 92
    Coconut-Tomato Seafood
        Curry, 148–149
    Creamy Summer
        Zoodles, 134
    Cucumber Green
        Smoothie, 65
    Kale-Mixed Vegetable
        Salad, 98–99
    Open-Faced Egg Sandwiches
        on Kale, 78–79
    Pesto-Kale Salad, 96
    Scrambled Egg and Kale, 74
    Simple Falafel, 126–127
    Tomato-Baked Bass, 159
    Vanilla-Kale Smoothie, 66
    Veggie Breakfast Skillet, 73
Kettlebells, 20–21
Kohlrabi
    Curried Kohlrabi, 118–119

L
Leafy greens. See also specific
    about, 14–15
    Avocado-Tangerine Salad, 97
    Radish and Egg Salad, 95

LEAP protocol, 28
Leeks
    Asparagus with Shallots, 125
    Chicken-Veggie
        Broth, 206–207
    Turkey, Leek, and Pumpkin
        Casserole, 174
Lemons and lemon juice
    Asparagus with Shallots, 125
    Avocado-Chickpea
        Tabbouleh, 129
    Avocado-Citrus Soup, 85
    Baked Sole with Parsley
        Pistou, 158
    Basil-Tomato Salad with
        Herb Vinaigrette, 93
    Chicken Breasts with
        Raspberry Sauce, 170–171
    Classic Gremolata Sauce, 210
    Cold Cucumber-Dill Soup, 83
    Creamy Coconut Yogurt, 214
    Curried Cabbage Salad, 94
    Garlic Shrimp and
        Vegetables, 140
    Greek Fish Stew, 144–145
    Harissa-Rubbed Bass, 151
    Mediterranean Spaghetti
        Squash, 111
    Mussels in Coconut
        Broth, 138
    Radish and Chicken
        Salad-Stuffed Endive, 110
    Roasted Eggplant Dip, 102
    Roasted Sole with
        Vegetables, Garlic, and
        Sunflower Seeds, 146
    Roasted Trout with
        Fennel, 157
    Sesame-Lemon Dressing, 211
    Simple Falafel, 126–127
    Spice-Rubbed Flounder with
        Citrus Salsa, 154–155
    Thyme-Baked Artichokes, 114

Lettuce
    Lettuce Spring Rolls, 103
Limes and lime juice
    Asian Spinach Salad with
        Almond Dressing, 92
    Baked Tilapia with
        Blueberry-Avocado
        Salsa, 163
    Coconut Milk-Braised
        Chicken, 173
    Creamy Summer
        Zoodles, 134
    Easy Chicken Pad
        Thai, 168–169
    Lime Cheesecake, 198
    Refreshing Gazpacho, 82
    Roasted Venison Leg, 180
    Turkey-Zucchini Noodle
        Salad, 90
Lutein, 15
Lycopene, 15

M

Meal plans
    fighting brain fog, 54–56
    gaining energy, 51–53
    pain management, 48–50
    promoting healthy
        digestion, 57–59
Meats. See also Pork
    Acorn Squash Lamb
        Gratin, 184–185
    Lamb-Vegetable
        Stew, 182–183
    Mustard-Crusted
        Venison, 181
    Roasted Venison Leg, 180
    shopping for, 39
Mediator release test, 28
Medications, 16–17
Mental health, 19
Migrating motor complex
    (MMC), 8

Mindful eating, 34–35
Minerals, 9, 16–17
Mint
    Avocado-Chickpea
        Tabbouleh, 129
    Roasted Venison Leg, 180
Mushrooms
    Beef Chow Mein, 188–189
    Chicken with Wild
        Mushrooms, 167
    Portobello Mushroom–Baked
        Eggs, 128
    Scrambled Egg and Kale, 74
    Turkey Chili, 178
    Turkey Stroganoff, 175
Mussels
    Greek Fish Stew, 144–145
    Mussels in Coconut
        Broth, 138

N

Neurotransmitters, 4–5
Nonreactive foods, 28
Nut-Free recipes
    about, 45
    Avocado-Chickpea
        Tabbouleh, 129
    Avocado-Citrus Soup, 85
    Avocado-Tangerine Salad, 97
    Balsamic-Braised Onions, 117
    Basil-Tomato Salad with
        Herb Vinaigrette, 93
    Beef Pot Roast with
        Vegetables, 190
    Bell Pepper-Asparagus
        Frittata, 76
    Blueberry Jam, 215
    Cajun Scallops, 139
    Caramelized Onion and
        Spinach Omelet, 71
    Chicken Breasts with
        Raspberry Sauce, 170–171
    Chicken Cacciatore, 172
    Chicken Chili Soup, 89

Nut-Free recipes (continued)
Chicken-Veggie
Broth, 206–207
Chicken with Wild
Mushrooms, 167
Chickpea Basil-Stuffed
Peppers, 124
Classic Gremolata Sauce, 210
Creamy Chocolate
Mousse, 196
Creamy Saffron Chicken, 166
Creamy Summer
Zoodles, 134
Crispy Baked Parsnip
Fries, 104
Fresh Summer Salad, 91
Garlic Shrimp and
Vegetables, 140
Gingered Asparagus, 121
Glorious Carrot Soup, 88
Greek Fish Stew, 144–145
Harissa-Rubbed Bass, 151
Herb and Roasted Red
Pepper Pesto, 208
Homemade Sauerkraut, 120
Kale-Mixed Vegetable
Salad, 98–99
Lamb-Vegetable
Stew, 182–183
Lettuce Spring Rolls, 103
Lime Cheesecake, 198
Mediterranean Spaghetti
Squash, 111
Open-Faced Egg Sandwiches
on Kale, 78–79
Panfried Tilapia
with Compound
Butter, 152–153
Pesto-Kale Salad, 96
Pork Tenderloin with
Caramelized Onions, 179
Portobello Mushroom–Baked
Eggs, 128

Pretty Pickled
Jalapeños, 112–113
Pumpkin, Turkey, and Swiss
Chard Hash, 72
Radish and Egg Salad, 95
Refreshing Gazpacho, 82
Rich Beef Broth, 204–205
Roasted Bell Pepper
Trout, 160–161
Roasted Cauliflower-Broccoli
Soup, 87
Roasted Eggplant Dip, 102
Roasted Sole with
Vegetables, Garlic, and
Sunflower Seeds, 146
Roasted Vegetables with
Thyme, 130
Roasted Venison Leg, 180
Sausage with Celeriac
Latkes, 75
Scrambled Egg and Kale, 74
Shrimp Egg Foo
Young, 142–143
Simple Pork Sausage, 77
Southwestern Cauliflower
Rice, 116
Spice-Rubbed Flounder with
Citrus Salsa, 154–155
Sweet Potato and Chickpea
Sauté, 132–133
Thyme-Baked Artichokes, 114
Tomato-Baked Bass, 159
Tomato-Jalapeño Soup, 86
Turkey Chili, 178
Turkey, Leek, and Pumpkin
Casserole, 174
Turkey Shepherd's
Pie, 176–177
Turkey Stroganoff, 175
Veggie Breakfast Skillet, 73
Versatile Barbecue Rub, 212
Nuts and seeds. See specific

O
Olives, Kalamata
Basil-Tomato Salad with
Herb Vinaigrette, 93
Chickpea Basil-Stuffed
Peppers, 124
Greek Fish Stew, 144–145
Roasted Eggplant Dip, 102
Onions
Balsamic-Braised Onions, 117
Caramelized Onion and
Spinach Omelet, 71
Pork Tenderloin with
Caramelized Onions, 179
Oranges and orange juice
Avocado-Tangerine Salad, 97
Citrus-Berry Ambrosia, 195
Coconut Milk-Turmeric
Smoothie, 68
Easy Chicken Pad
Thai, 168–169
Orange-Pistachio Bass, 147
Panfried Tilapia
with Compound
Butter, 152–153
Sole with Ginger-Wasabi
Glaze, 162
Spice-Rubbed Flounder with
Citrus Salsa, 154–155
Oregano
Asparagus with Shallots, 125
Chicken Cacciatore, 172
Italian-Style Meatballs, 191
Kale-Mixed Vegetable
Salad, 98–99
Mediterranean Spaghetti
Squash, 111
Orange-Pistachio Bass, 147
Roasted Eggplant Dip, 102
Traditional Herbed
Meatloaf, 186
Winter Vegetable Stew, 135
Zucchini Pasta with Beef and
Eggplant Sauce, 187
Oxidative stress, 9

P

Pain, chronic, 7–8, 42–43
  Emotional aspect of, 43
  Sensory aspect of, 42–43
Paleo-Friendly recipes
  about, 45
  Almond-Sesame Seed
    Balls, 107
  Asparagus with Shallots, 125
  Avocado-Tangerine Salad, 97
  Baked Sole with Parsley
    Pistou, 158
  Baked Tilapia with
    Blueberry-Avocado
    Salsa, 163
  Balsamic-Braised Onions, 117
  Basil-Tomato Salad with
    Herb Vinaigrette, 93
  Beef Pot Roast with
    Vegetables, 190
  Cajun Scallops, 139
  Chicken Breasts with
    Raspberry Sauce, 170–171
  Chicken Cacciatore, 172
  Chicken-Veggie
    Broth, 206–207
  Chicken with Wild
    Mushrooms, 167
  Chopped Veggie Bowl, 131
  Classic Gremolata Sauce, 210
  Coconut Milk-Turmeric
    Smoothie, 68
  Coconut-Tomato Seafood
    Curry, 148–149
  Cold Cucumber-Dill Soup, 83
  Crispy Baked Parsnip
    Fries, 104
  Cucumber Green
    Smoothie, 65
  Curried Kohlrabi, 118–119
  Fresh Summer Salad, 91
  Garlic Shrimp and
    Vegetables, 140
  Gingered Asparagus, 121
  Greek Fish Stew, 144–145

  Harissa-Rubbed Bass, 151
  Herb and Roasted Red
    Pepper Pesto, 208
  Homemade Almond
    Milk, 213
  Homemade Sauerkraut, 120
  Italian-Style Meatballs, 191
  Kale-Mixed Vegetable
    Salad, 98–99
  Lamb-Vegetable
    Stew, 182–183
  Lettuce Spring Rolls, 103
  Mediterranean Spaghetti
    Squash, 111
  Mussels in Coconut
    Broth, 138
  Mustard-Crusted
    Venison, 181
  Open-Faced Egg Sandwiches
    on Kale, 78–79
  Orange-Pistachio Bass, 147
  Panfried Tilapia
    with Compound
    Butter, 152–153
  Pesto-Kale Salad, 96
  Pork Tenderloin with
    Caramelized Onions, 179
  Portobello Mushroom–Baked
    Eggs, 128
  Pumpkin, Turkey, and Swiss
    Chard Hash, 72
  Rich Beef Broth, 204–205
  Roasted Bell Pepper
    Trout, 160–161
  Roasted Eggplant Dip, 102
  Roasted Sole with
    Vegetables, Garlic, and
    Sunflower Seeds, 146
  Roasted Vegetables with
    Thyme, 130
  Sausage with Celeriac
    Latkes, 75
  Sesame-Lemon Dressing, 211
  Shrimp Egg Foo
    Young, 142–143
  Simple Pork Sausage, 77

  Southwestern Cauliflower
    Rice, 116
  Spice-Rubbed Flounder with
    Citrus Salsa, 154–155
  Sweet Potato-Brussels
    Sprouts Toss, 115
  Thai Coconut Milk Soup, 84
  Thyme-Baked Artichokes, 114
  Tomato-Baked Bass, 159
  Tomato-Jalapeño Soup, 86
  Trout-Pumpkin Patties, 141
  Turkey, Leek, and Pumpkin
    Casserole, 174
  Vanilla-Kale Smoothie, 66
  Versatile Barbecue Rub, 212
  Zucchini Pasta with Beef and
    Eggplant Sauce, 187
Pantry staples, 36–38
Parsley
  Acorn Squash Lamb
    Gratin, 184–185
  Avocado-Chickpea
    Tabbouleh, 129
  Baked Sole with Parsley
    Pistou, 158
  Basil-Tomato Salad with
    Herb Vinaigrette, 93
  Chicken Cacciatore, 172
  Chicken-Veggie
    Broth, 206–207
  Classic Gremolata Sauce, 210
  Fresh Summer Salad, 91
  Glorious Carrot Soup, 88
  Greek Fish Stew, 144–145
  Herb and Roasted Red
    Pepper Pesto, 208
  Italian-Style Meatballs, 191
  Portobello Mushroom–Baked
    Eggs, 128
  Radish and Chicken
    Salad-Stuffed Endive, 110
  Simple Pork Sausage, 77
  Traditional Herbed
    Meatloaf, 186
  Turkey Stroganoff, 175

Parsnips
  Crispy Baked Parsnip
    Fries, 104
  Curried Cabbage Salad, 94
  Lamb-Vegetable
    Stew, 182–183
  Roasted Sole with
    Vegetables, Garlic, and
    Sunflower Seeds, 146
  Sweet Potato and Chickpea
    Sauté, 132–133
  Winter Vegetable Stew, 135
Pecans
  Nut-Chili Crackers, 106
  Sweet Potato-Brussels
    Sprouts Toss, 115
  Sweet Potato Pudding, 197
Physiologic diet, 11
Pine nuts
  Pesto-Kale Salad, 96
Pistachios
  Almond-Sesame Seed
    Balls, 107
  Chocolate-Pistachio
    Shake, 64
  Mustard-Crusted
    Venison, 181
  Orange-Pistachio Bass, 147
Pork. See also Bacon
  Pork Tenderloin with
    Caramelized Onions, 179
  Sausage with Celeriac
    Latkes, 75
  Simple Pork Sausage, 77
  Traditional Herbed
    Meatloaf, 186
Posture work, 21
Poultry. See Chicken; Turkey
Progesterone, 5–7
Pumpkin
  Pumpkin, Turkey, and Swiss
    Chard Hash, 72
  Trout-Pumpkin Patties, 141
  Turkey, Leek, and Pumpkin
    Casserole, 174

Pumpkin seeds
  Herb and Roasted Red
    Pepper Pesto, 208
  Sweet Potato and Chickpea
    Sauté, 132–133

R

Radicchio
  Radish and Egg Salad, 95
Radishes
  Kale-Mixed Vegetable
    Salad, 98–99
  Radish and Chicken
    Salad-Stuffed Endive, 110
  Radish and Egg Salad, 95
Rapini
  Avocado-Tangerine Salad, 97
Raspberries
  Berry Brown Betty, 199
  Chicken Breasts with
    Raspberry Sauce, 170–171
Reactive foods, 28
Rebounding, 20
Ricotta cheese
  Caramelized Onion and
    Spinach Omelet, 71
Rosemary
  Lamb-Vegetable
    Stew, 182–183
  Mustard-Crusted
    Venison, 181

S

Saffron
  Coconut Milk-Baked
    Catfish, 156
  Creamy Saffron Chicken, 166
Scallions
  Asian Spinach Salad with
    Almond Dressing, 92
  Avocado-Chickpea
    Tabbouleh, 129

Beef Chow Mein, 188–189
Bell Pepper-Asparagus
  Frittata, 76
Chicken Chili Soup, 89
Easy Chicken Pad
  Thai, 168–169
Garlic Shrimp and
  Vegetables, 140
Mediterranean Spaghetti
  Squash, 111
Mussels in Coconut
  Broth, 138
Pesto-Kale Salad, 96
Radish and Chicken
  Salad-Stuffed Endive, 110
Roasted Bell Pepper
  Trout, 160–161
Roasted Vegetables with
  Thyme, 130
Shrimp Egg Foo
  Young, 142–143
Spice-Rubbed Flounder with
  Citrus Salsa, 154–155
Sweet Potato and Chickpea
  Sauté, 132–133
Trout-Pumpkin Patties, 141
Turkey Chili, 178
Veggie Breakfast Skillet, 73
Scallops
  Cajun Scallops, 139
Serotonin, 4–5, 8–10
Sesame seeds
  Almond-Sesame Seed
    Balls, 107
  Beef Chow Mein, 188–189
  Turkey-Zucchini Noodle
    Salad, 90
Shallots
  Asparagus with Shallots, 125
  Chicken Breasts with
    Raspberry Sauce, 170–171
  Orange-Pistachio Bass, 147
Shopping guide, 38–39

Shrimp
 Coconut-Tomato Seafood
  Curry, 148–149
 Garlic Shrimp and
  Vegetables, 140
 Greek Fish Stew, 144–145
 Shrimp Egg Foo
  Young, 142–143
Sleep, 10, 19
Sleep apnea, 19
Sole
 Baked Sole with Parsley
  Pistou, 158
 Roasted Sole with
  Vegetables, Garlic, and
  Sunflower Seeds, 146
 Sole with Ginger-Wasabi
  Glaze, 162
Spinach
 Asian Spinach Salad with
  Almond Dressing, 92
 Caramelized Onion and
  Spinach Omelet, 71
 Fresh Summer Salad, 91
 Greek Fish Stew, 144–145
 Portobello Mushroom–Baked
  Eggs, 128
 Winter Vegetable Stew, 135
Spinal fluid, 5
Squash. See also Zucchini
 Acorn Squash Lamb
  Gratin, 184–185
 Easy Chicken Pad
  Thai, 168–169
 Mediterranean Spaghetti
  Squash, 111
 Roasted Vegetables with
  Thyme, 130
 Turkey Chili, 178
Strawberries
 Citrus-Berry Ambrosia, 195
Stress, 7, 44
Substance P, 5
Sunflower seeds
 Avocado-Tangerine Salad, 97
 Chopped Veggie Bowl, 131

Grapefruit-Yogurt
 Smoothie, 69
Kale-Mixed Vegetable
 Salad, 98–99
Roasted Sole with
 Vegetables, Garlic, and
 Sunflower Seeds, 146
Sweet potatoes
 Beef Pot Roast with
  Vegetables, 190
 Lamb-Vegetable
  Stew, 182–183
 Portobello Mushroom–Baked
  Eggs, 128
 Sweet Potato and Chickpea
  Sauté, 132–133
 Sweet Potato-Brussels
  Sprouts Toss, 115
 Sweet Potato Pudding, 197
 Thai Coconut Milk Soup, 84
 Turkey Shepherd's
  Pie, 176–177
 Veggie Breakfast Skillet, 73
 Winter Vegetable Stew, 135
Swimming, 21
Swiss chard
 Chopped Veggie Bowl, 131
 Pumpkin, Turkey, and Swiss
  Chard Hash, 72
 Roasted Sole with
  Vegetables, Garlic, and
  Sunflower Seeds, 146
Symptom tracking, 30–33, 44

T

Tahini
 Sesame-Lemon Dressing, 211
 Simple Falafel, 126–127
Tangerines
 Avocado-Tangerine Salad, 97
Tannins, 15
Thyme
 Chicken-Veggie
  Broth, 206–207

Mustard-Crusted
 Venison, 181
Panfried Tilapia
 with Compound
 Butter, 152–153
Pork Tenderloin with
 Caramelized Onions, 179
Pretty Pickled
 Jalapeños, 112–113
Pumpkin, Turkey, and Swiss
 Chard Hash, 72
Rich Beef Broth, 204–205
Roasted Vegetables with
 Thyme, 130
Sesame-Lemon Dressing, 211
Thyme-Baked Artichokes, 114
Turkey, Leek, and Pumpkin
 Casserole, 174
Turkey Shepherd's
 Pie, 176–177
Turkey Stroganoff, 175
Tilapia
 Baked Tilapia with
  Blueberry-Avocado
  Salsa, 163
 Panfried Tilapia
  with Compound
  Butter, 152–153
Tomatoes
 Acorn Squash Lamb
  Gratin, 184–185
 Avocado-Chickpea
  Tabbouleh, 129
 Avocado-Citrus Soup, 85
 Basil-Tomato Salad with
  Herb Vinaigrette, 93
 Bell Pepper-Asparagus
  Frittata, 76
 Chicken Cacciatore, 172
 Chickpea Basil-Stuffed
  Peppers, 124
 Coconut-Tomato Seafood
  Curry, 148–149
 Fresh Summer Salad, 91
 Greek Fish Stew, 144–145

Tomatoes *(continued)*
Kale-Mixed Vegetable
Salad, 98–99
Lamb-Vegetable
Stew, 182–183
Mediterranean Spaghetti
Squash, 111
Open-Faced Egg Sandwiches
on Kale, 78–79
Refreshing Gazpacho, 82
Southwestern Cauliflower
Rice, 116
Tomato-Baked Bass, 159
Tomato-Jalapeño Soup, 86
Turkey Chili, 178
Winter Vegetable Stew, 135
Zucchini Pasta with Beef and
Eggplant Sauce, 187
Tomatoes, sun-dried
Chicken Cacciatore, 172
Harissa-Rubbed Bass, 151
Tomato-Jalapeño Soup, 86
Trout
Roasted Bell Pepper
Trout, 160–161
Roasted Trout with
Fennel, 157
Trout-Pumpkin Patties, 141
Turkey
Pumpkin, Turkey, and Swiss
Chard Hash, 72
Turkey Chili, 178
Turkey, Leek, and Pumpkin
Casserole, 174
Turkey Shepherd's
Pie, 176–177
Turkey Stroganoff, 175
Turkey-Zucchini Noodle
Salad, 90

shopping for, 38–39
Vegetarian recipes
about, 45
Almond-Sesame Seed
Balls, 107
Asian Spinach Salad with
Almond Dressing, 92
Asparagus with Shallots, 125
Avocado-Chickpea
Tabbouleh, 129
Avocado-Tangerine Salad, 97
Balsamic-Braised Onions, 117
Basil-Tomato Salad with
Herb Vinaigrette, 93
Bell Pepper-Asparagus
Frittata, 76
Blueberry-Almond
Scones, 108–109
Blueberry Jam, 215
Caramelized Onion and
Spinach Omelet, 71
Chickpea Basil-Stuffed
Peppers, 124
Chocolate-Almond
Spread, 209
Chopped Veggie Bowl, 131
Cinnamon Cheesecake
Smoothie, 67
Citrus-Berry Ambrosia, 195
Classic Gremolata Sauce, 210
Creamy Chocolate
Mousse, 196
Creamy Coconut Yogurt, 214
Creamy Summer
Zoodles, 134
Crispy Baked Parsnip
Fries, 104
Curried Cabbage Salad, 94
Curried Kohlrabi, 118–119
Dark Chocolate Sheet
Cake, 200–201
Ginger-Coconut Cookies, 105
Gingered Asparagus, 121
Grapefruit-Yogurt
Smoothie, 69

Herb and Roasted Red
Pepper Pesto, 208
Homemade Almond
Milk, 213
Homemade Sauerkraut, 120
Kale-Mixed Vegetable
Salad, 98–99
Lettuce Spring Rolls, 103
Mediterranean Spaghetti
Squash, 111
Mixed Nut Porridge, 70
Nut-Chili Crackers, 106
Pesto-Kale Salad, 96
Portobello Mushroom–Baked
Eggs, 128
Pretty Pickled
Jalapeños, 112–113
Radish and Egg Salad, 95
Refreshing Gazpacho, 82
Roasted Eggplant Dip, 102
Roasted Vegetables with
Thyme, 130
Scrambled Egg and Kale, 74
Sesame-Lemon Dressing, 211
Simple Falafel, 126–127
Sweet Potato and Chickpea
Sauté, 132–133
Sweet Potato-Brussels
Sprouts Toss, 115
Sweet Potato Pudding, 197
Thyme-Baked Artichokes, 114
Veggie Breakfast Skillet, 73
Versatile Barbecue Rub, 212
Winter Vegetable Stew, 135
Vitamins, 16–17

W

Walking intervals, 21
Walnuts
Asparagus with Shallots, 125
Baked Tilapia with
Blueberry-Avocado
Salsa, 163
Curried Kohlrabi, 118–119

N

Vagus nerve, 4
Vegetables. *See also specific*
cruciferous, 15
nightshades, 15

Wasabi
  Sole with Ginger-Wasabi
    Glaze, 162
Whitefish
  Coconut-Tomato Seafood
    Curry, 148–149
  Greek Fish Stew, 144–145

Y

Yogurt
  Avocado-Citrus Soup, 85
  Chicken Chili Soup, 89
  Cinnamon Cheesecake
    Smoothie, 67
  Citrus-Berry Ambrosia, 195

Creamy Saffron Chicken, 166
Curried Cabbage Salad, 94
Grapefruit-Yogurt
  Smoothie, 69
Mixed Nut Porridge, 70
Radish and Chicken
  Salad-Stuffed Endive, 110
Refreshing Gazpacho, 82
Turkey Chili, 178

Z

Zucchini
  Chicken with Wild
    Mushrooms, 167

Creamy Summer
  Zoodles, 134
Easy Chicken Pad
  Thai, 168–169
Fresh Summer Salad, 91
Roasted Bell Pepper
  Trout, 160–161
Roasted Vegetables with
  Thyme, 130
Tomato-Baked Bass, 159
Turkey-Zucchini Noodle
  Salad, 90
Veggie Breakfast Skillet, 73
Zucchini Pasta with Beef and
  Eggplant Sauce, 187

ACKNOWLEDGMENTS

To Roger and Marie Moulton, who taught me never to be afraid to use my voice for honesty and truth. To Dr. Christy Kesslering, Dr. Mark Nelson, Dr. Azlan Tariq, Dr. Kathleen Collins, and all the medical professionals who believe in the power of nutrition and practice with science, ethics, and compassion. To my patients and clients for sharing your journeys with me and entrusting me with your nutrition care.

ABOUT THE AUTHOR

Kathleen Standafer is a Registered Dietitian Nutritionist, Board-Certified Nutrition Support Clinician, and Certified LEAP Therapist. She received her bachelor of science in dietetics from Iowa State University and master's degree in nutrition from the University of Central Oklahoma. She has published several articles for Livestrong and *SF Gate* and has had numerous TV and radio appearances. She has lived and worked in Iowa, Colorado, Missouri, Texas, Illinois, and Germany and has treated all ages and a spectrum of medical conditions. Kathleen uses a root-cause approach and enjoys questioning conventional nutrition practices. Kathleen serves as Dietetic Student Preceptor and Instructor at Dominican University and runs a private practice at a medical fitness clinic in Naperville, Illinois. Kathleen's philosophy is based on optimizing health by balancing insulin, oxidative stress, inflammation, and natural circadian rhythms.

CPSIA information can be obtained
at www.ICGtesting.com
Printed in the USA
BVOW10s0820070717

488702BV00001BA/1/P